Advances in Hyaluronic Acid Filler Injections

Won Lee

Advances in Hyaluronic Acid Filler Injections

Springer

Won Lee
Yonsei E1 Plastic Surgery Clinic
Anyang, Kyonggi-do, Korea (Republic of)

ISBN 978-981-97-6527-0 ISBN 978-981-97-6528-7 (eBook)
https://doi.org/10.1007/978-981-97-6528-7

This Springer imprint is published by the registered company Springer Nature Singapore Pte Ltd.
The registered company address is: 152 Beach Road, #21-01/04 Gateway East, Singapore 189721, Singapore

Preface

Hyaluronic acid in conjunction with botulinum toxin is considered a remarkable substance in the field of medical esthetics. Hyaluronic acid fillers, formulated by crosslinking hyaluronic acid, have gained popularity among doctors worldwide owing to their biodegradability advantage. Although many aspects of hyaluronic acid fillers remain unknown, new information is being gradually discovered. Moreover, safer procedures are continually introduced, thanks to the advancements of hyaluronic acid filler products and various scientific technologies.

Since my previous publication of a book on the matter, I have published over 65 research papers wherein a majority aimed to shed light on the various scientific aspects related to hyaluronic acid fillers. As a researcher and an author, I have conducted numerous experiments. While not all being perfect, I believe that I could amalgamate my understanding thus far to provide some key guidelines on the side-effect of blindness caused by hyaluronic acid fillers in this book.

We first discuss the importance of the composition of the fillers. Hyaluronic acid fillers should be produced solely from hyaluronic acid and a crosslinking agent. However, the impurities and insufficiently crosslinked agents that are inevitably introduced during the manufacturing process cause significant interference. Through my multiple visits to Korea Advanced Institute of Science and Technology (KAIST) and conducting experiments one by one, I experienced the joy of discovering the specifics of a key point that I had wanted to reveal for years, particularly through my direct nuclear magnetic resonance (NMR) experiments. This information is deeply discussed in this book.

Although safety concerns remain, ultrasound-guided injection of fillers, which allows the direct visualization of blood vessels, is considered a safer method. Therefore, I have included numerous cases, starting from the basics of the procedure. This book has been written with the most up-to-date information, aiming to revisit the guidelines on safety.

I would like to express my gratitude to Mr. Yoon Yeo Myeung, CEO of Joonghun Pharmaceuticals, for supporting the publication of this book. I extend my appreciation to my daughters, Seunghyun and Hyunji, for their unwavering support. And as always, I give my thanks to Jung Youn with love.

Above all, I dedicate this book to my father, Lee Jeong Yoon, who continues to bless us from heaven, and my mother-in-law, Lee Hyang Ran, who is also present only in spirit, for being an irreplaceable pillar in our lives for over 25 years.

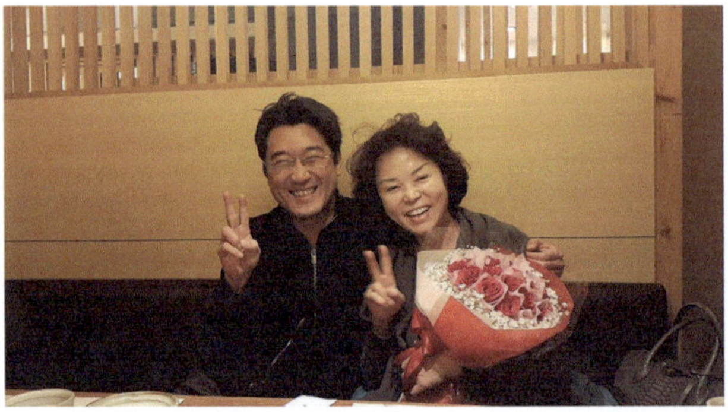

Anyang, Kyonggi-do, Korea (Republic of) Won Lee
April 2024

Contents

Anatomy of the Face for Hyaluronic Acid Filler Injection

1

Contents

1.1 Introduction

The main purpose of filler injections is to restore facial volume. Thus, subcutaneous injections are most effective; yet the abundant vasculature in the subcutaneous layer is a key impediment. Therefore, identification of the basic arterial pathway is recommended. In this chapter we will discuss the arteries of the face and other basic facial anatomical structures.

1.2 Arteries of the Face

The important arteries of the faces (Fig. 1.1) and hyaluronic acid filler injection locations are as follows:

1.2.1 Internal Carotid Artery Territories

Supratrochlear artery	Glabellar frown line correction
Supraorbital artery	Forehead augmentation
Dorsal nasal artery	Nose augmentation

1.2.2 External Carotid Artery Territories

Facial artery	Nasolabial fold correction
Frontal branch of superficial temporal artery	Temple augmentation
Superior and inferior labial artery	Lip augmentation
Infraorbital artery	Anterior malar augmentation

W. Lee, *Advances in Hyaluronic Acid Filler Injections*,
https://doi.org/10.1007/978-981-97-6528-7_1

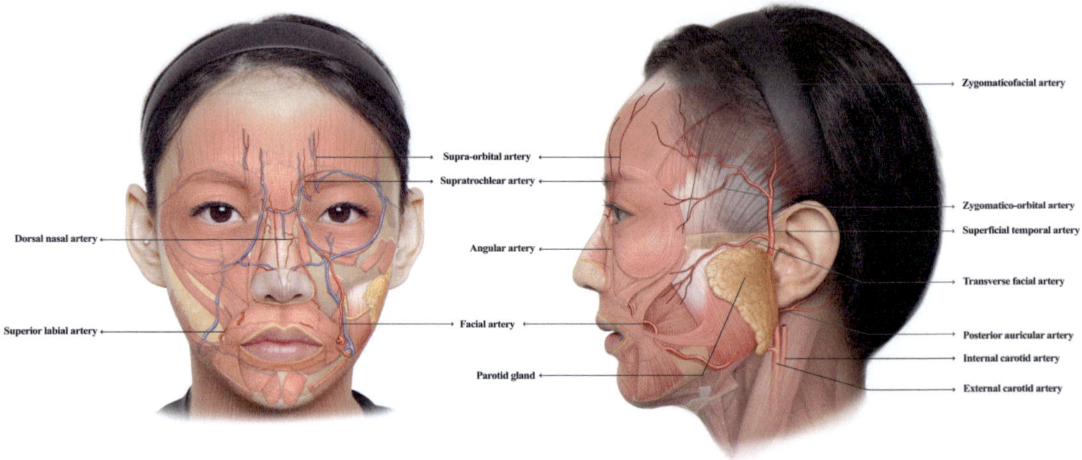

Fig. 1.1 Arteries of the face

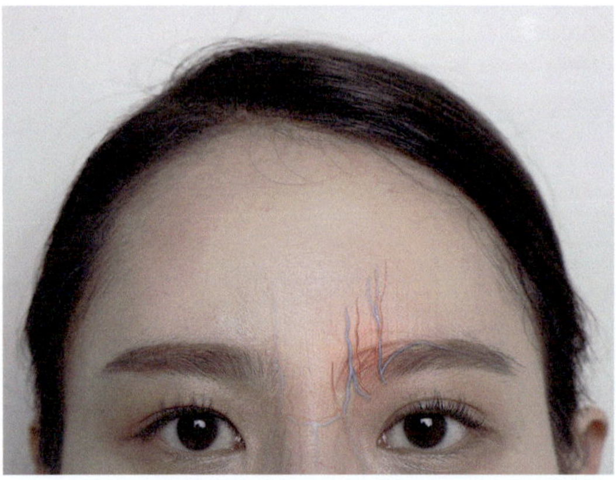

Fig. 1.2 Surface anatomy of supratrochlear artery

Vascular complications are the most tragic complications of hyaluronic acid filler injection. Therefore, the injector should be aware of the facial vasculature anatomy. However, the facial vasculature has individual patient variations; therefore, to make the filler injection procedure safer, Doppler ultrasound would be a safer option. We will discuss the arteries of the face by region and compare them with cadaveric and Doppler ultrasound images.

1.2.3 Supratrochlear Artery

The supratrochlear artery is important to be aware of when performing glabellar wrinkle corrections and forehead augmentation (Fig. 1.2).

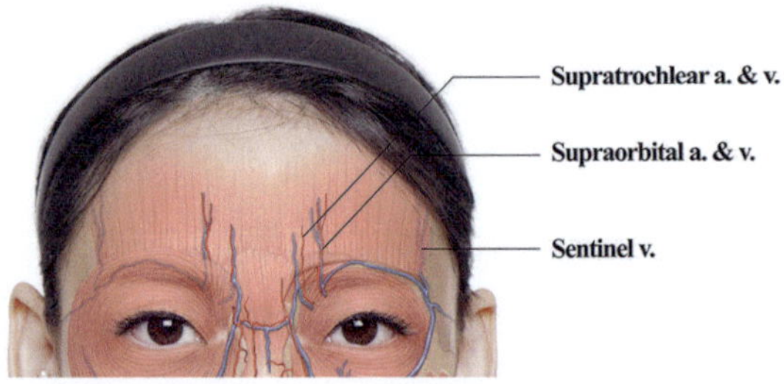

Fig. 1.3 Schematic diagram of supratrochlear artery and supraorbital artery

The artery divides into the superficial branch and deep branch, and forms an anastomosis with the supraorbital artery (Figs. 1.3 and 1.4). With Doppler ultrasound, one can detect whether the artery is deep or a superficial branch (Fig. 1.5).

The supratrochlear artery divides from the ophthalmic artery and medially perforates the orbital septum. It then runs toward the glabella area, superficially, but sometimes deeply [1]. Thus, Doppler ultrasonography is recommended to determine the location and depth of the supratrochlear artery before injection into the glabellar frown wrinkle line.

1.2.4 Frontal Branch of Superficial Temporal Artery

The frontal branch of the superficial temporal artery (FBrSTA) is located in the temple area and can complicate the injection site of the hyaluronic acid filler in the temple area (Fig. 1.6). The FBrSTA originates from the external carotid artery and is located in the lateral forehead area by one or more branches (Fig. 1.7). Cadaveric study describes that the FBrSTA is located at subcutaneous layer at 17.7 mm medially and 36.9 mm superiorly from the tragus (Fig. 1.8) [2]. However, there is always variation of the arterial pathway, and its relationship with the hairline is important [3]. Thus, Doppler ultrasonography is recommended to avoid this potential complication, as well (Fig. 1.9).

When Doppler ultrasound is performed, it is possible to detect the correlation between the FBrSTA location and the hairline. Some patients can visualize the FBrSTA and/or the anastomosis from the supraorbital artery because of the shallowing of the subcutaneous fat layer caused by the aging process. Thus, in some patients, arterial pulses can be detected by palpation. However, Doppler ultrasonography is recommended when palpation is undetectable. Doppler ultrasonography can be used to detect the location of the deep temporal artery. Temple augmentation by hyal-

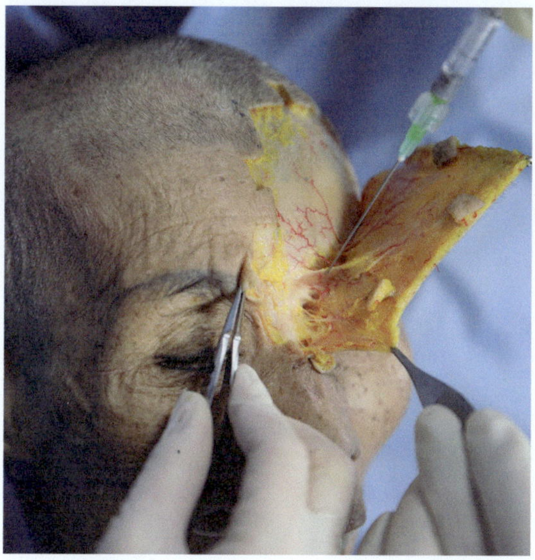

Fig. 1.4 Cadaveric dissection of the supratrochlear artery deep and superficial branches

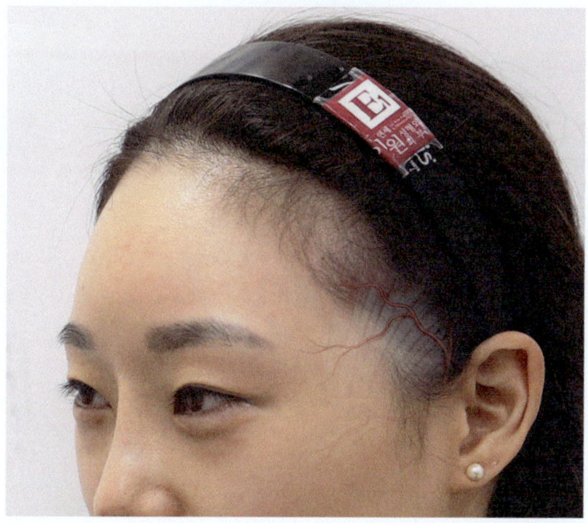

Fig. 1.6 Surface anatomy of the superficial temporal artery

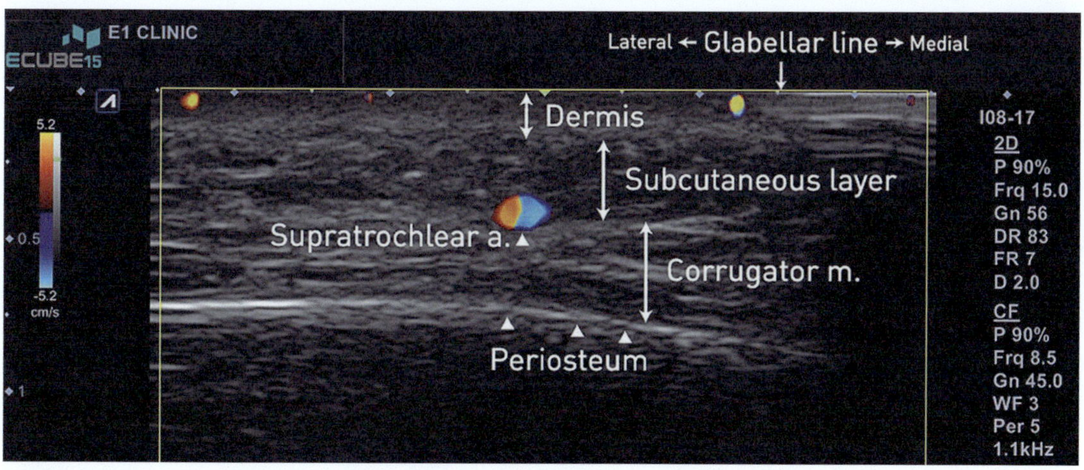

Fig. 1.5 Doppler ultrasound image of the supratrochlear artery

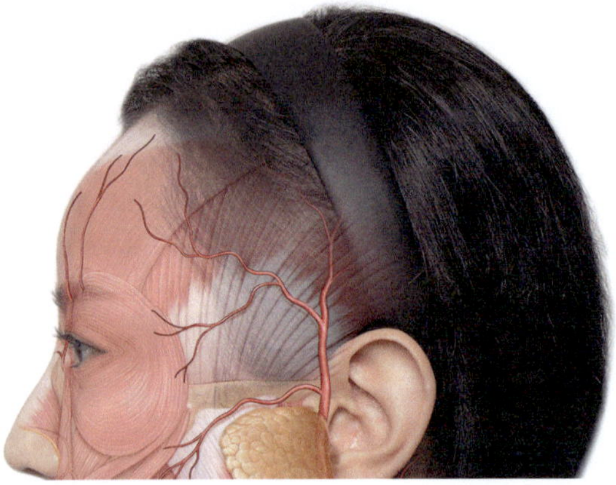

Fig. 1.7 Schematic diagram of the superficial temporal artery

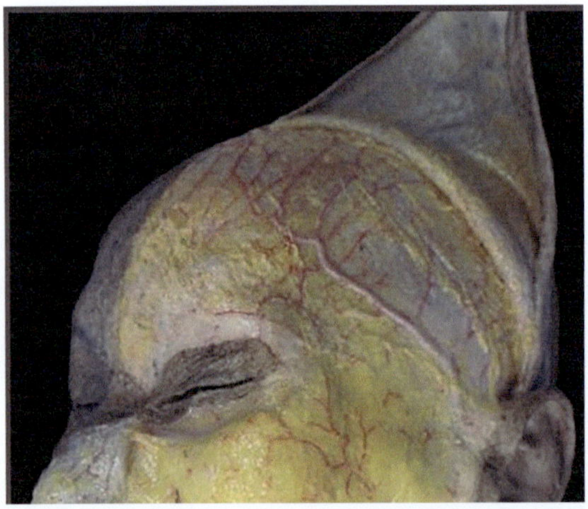

Fig. 1.8 Cadaveric finding of the FBrSTA

uronic acid filler injection technique is described in Chap. 4.

1.2.5 Dorsal Nasal Artery

The dorsal nasal artery is an important vessel for nose augmentation by hyaluronic acid filler injections. Usually, it is located in the radix subcutaneous layer, but many variations exist, such as the midline cross (Figs. 1.10 and 1.11). The artery is at the branch of the ophthalmic artery, one of the most critical arteries of the face to avoid (Fig. 1.12). Doppler ultrasound can be used to detect the dorsal nasal artery before the hyaluronic acid filler injection (Fig. 1.13).

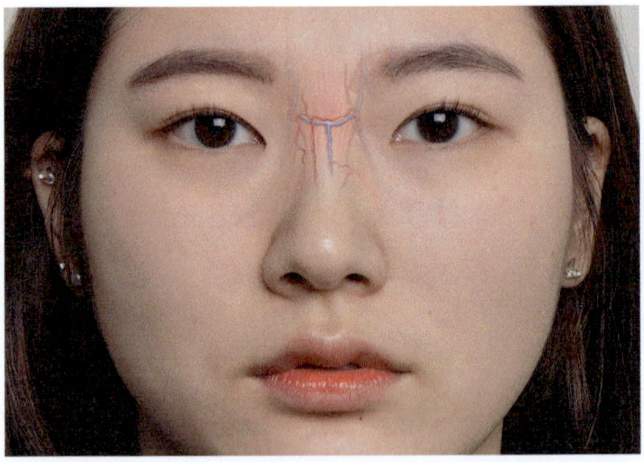

Fig. 1.10 Surface anatomy of dorsal nasal artery

Fig. 1.9 Doppler ultrasound finding of the FBrSTA and a deep temporal artery

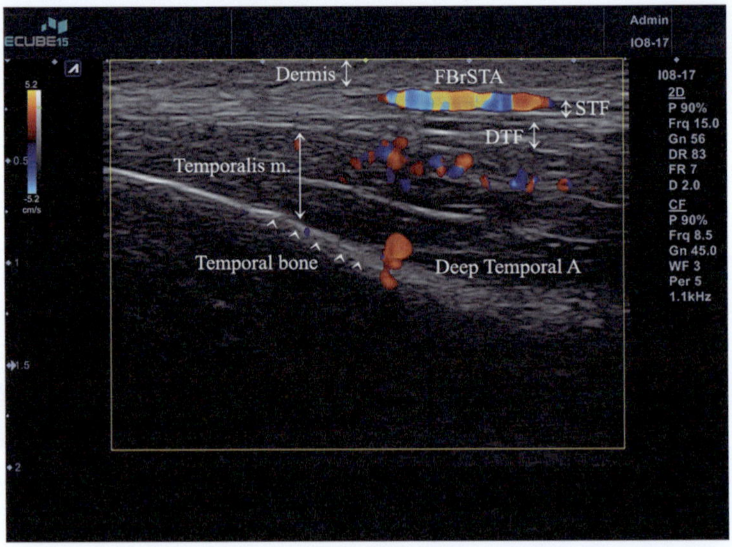

Usually, it is recommended to use a cannula when performing hyaluronic acid filler because of its safety, but there are many cases of ocular complications when nose augmentation by a cannula is used. The dorsal nasal artery tends to cross the midline [4]; thus, a 23G or 25G cannula can compromise the artery. The techniques of nose augmentation by hyaluronic acid fillers are described in Chap. 3.

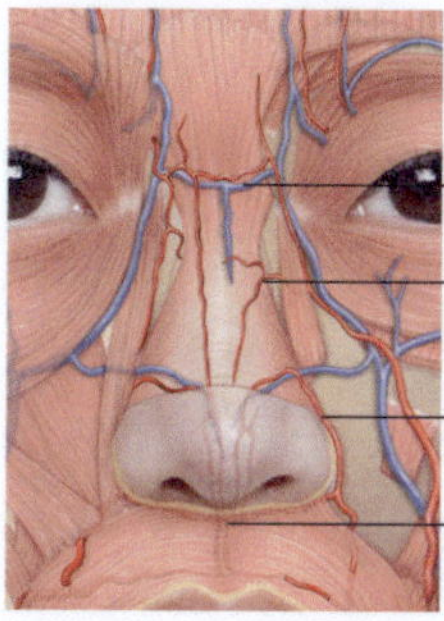

Fig. 1.11 Schematic diagram of the paranasal area

1.2.6 Facial Artery

The facial artery runs along the nasolabial fold area (Figs. 1.14 and 1.15). Cadaveric anatomy typically shows that the facial artery is located in the subcutaneous layer of the nasolabial fold area (Fig. 1.16). Doppler ultrasonography also showed a facial artery located in the subcutaneous layer (Fig. 1.17).

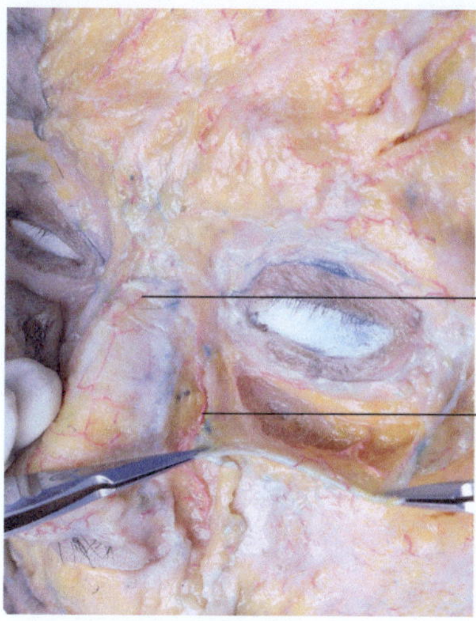

Fig. 1.12 Cadaveric anatomy of dorsal nasal artery anastomosis with the angular artery

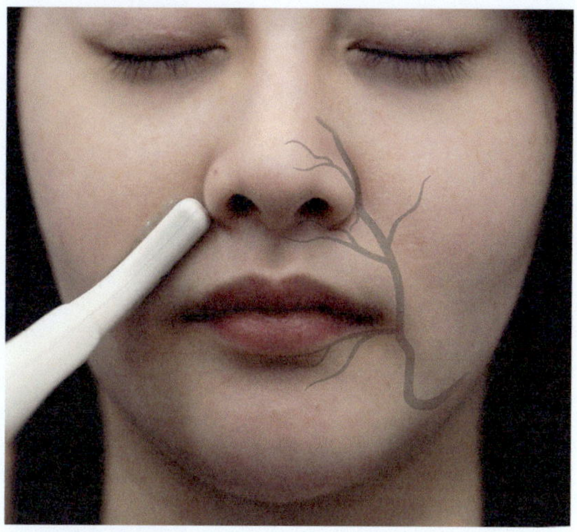

Fig. 1.14 Surface anatomy of the facial artery

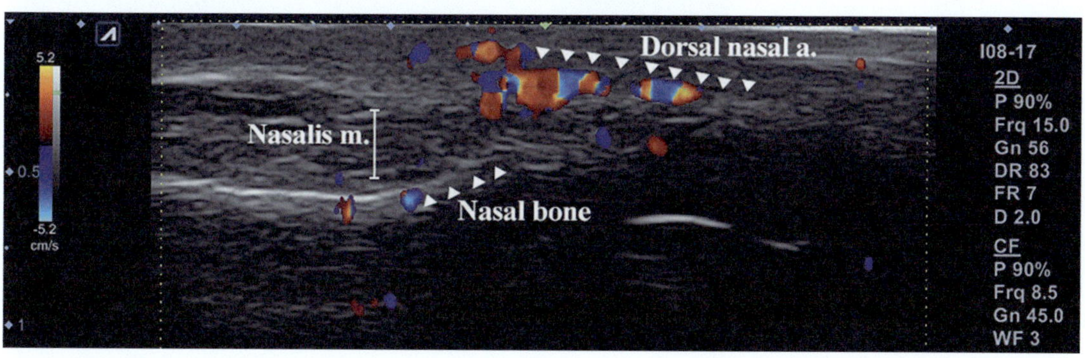

Fig. 1.13 Doppler ultrasound finding of the dorsal nasal artery

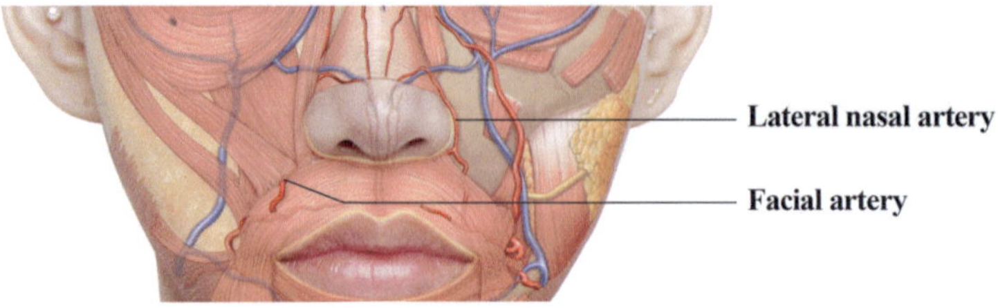

Fig. 1.15 Schematic anatomy of the facial artery

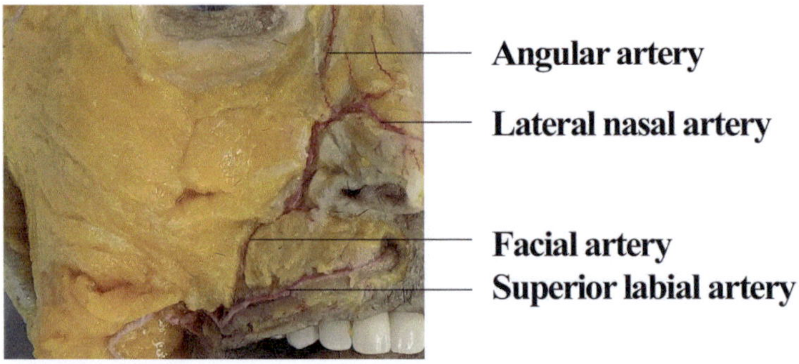

Fig. 1.16 Cadaveric anatomy of the facial artery

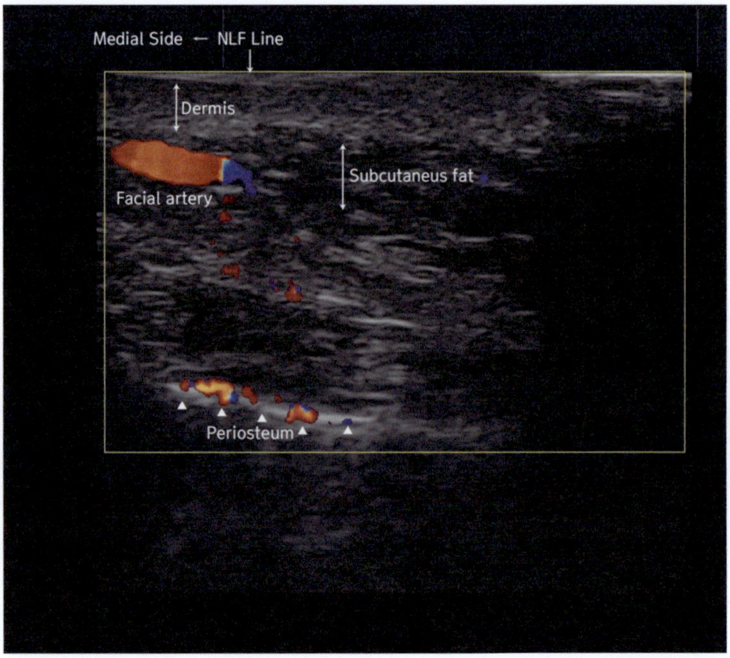

Fig. 1.17 Doppler ultrasound finding of facial artery reveals its location at the subcutaneous layer

However, the facial artery can run deep into the nasolabial fold. Its location can also be found directed toward the infraorbital foramen [5]. Thus, Doppler ultrasonography is recommended before injecting hyaluronic acid fillers to correct the nasolabial fold.

Understanding the location of the arteries of the face is critical when performing hyaluronic acid filler injections. However, as all the arterial variations cannot be estimated, Doppler ultrasound emerges as an important method to safely detect the arteries of the face. The Doppler ultrasound techniques will be discussed in Chaps. 3 and 4.

1.3 Muscles of the Face

Understanding facial muscles is important for the safe delivery of hyaluronic acid fillers under or over the facial muscles (Fig. 1.18). The anatomy should also be known because of the possible migration of hyaluronic acid fillers from the repetitive muscle contractions. When performing forehead augmentation with hyaluronic acid filler, botulinum toxin injection is recommended because of the repetitive contraction of the frontalis muscle. When temple augmentation is performed by hyaluronic acid fillers, considering the deeper or more superficial injection from the temporalis muscle becomes key. Hyaluronic acid filler is a viscoelastic material that can aggregate at one location due to repetitive muscle contraction; thus, understanding muscle anatomy becomes essential.

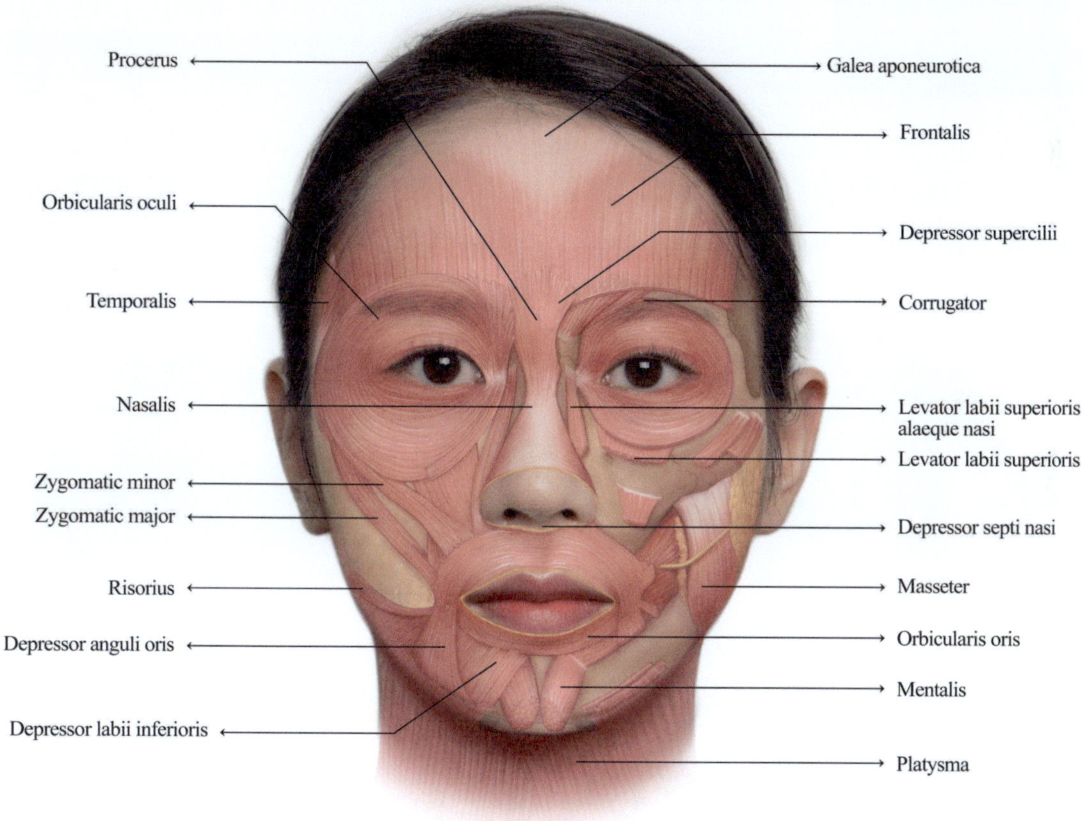

Fig. 1.18 Facial musculatures

1.4 Superficial and Deep Fat Compartments

An important aspect of the aging process is soft tissue descent and absorption of the fat compartment. Understanding the superficial and deep fat compartments can help fill the absorbed fat compartments (Fig. 1.19). Fat absorption differs depending on the facial region (Fig. 1.20).

Lateral cheek deflation can be observed in the early 40s and malar deflation in the 50s.

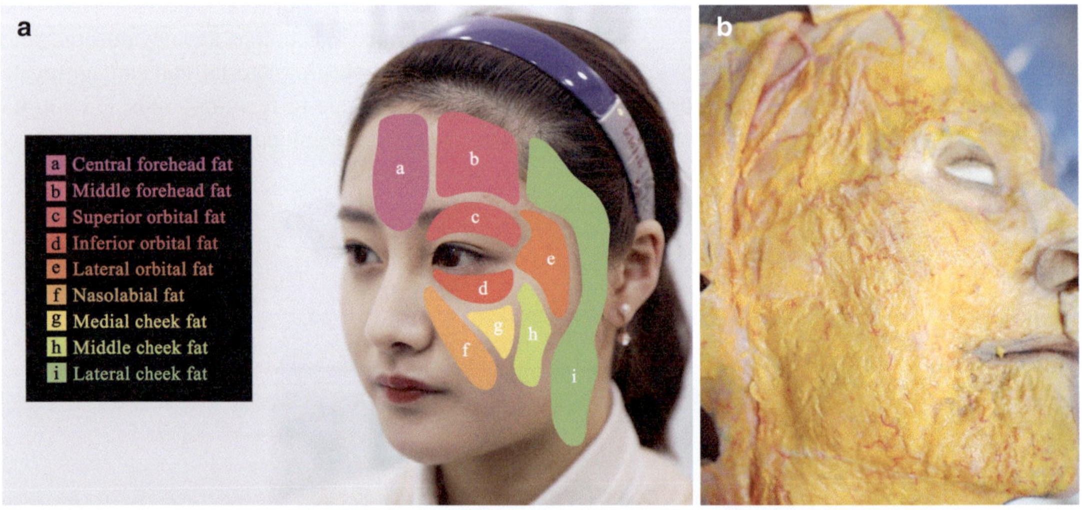
a
a Central forehead fat
b Middle forehead fat
c Superior orbital fat
d Inferior orbital fat
e Lateral orbital fat
f Nasolabial fat
g Medial cheek fat
h Middle cheek fat
i Lateral cheek fat
a
b
c
d
e
f
g
h
i
b

Fig. 1.19 Superficial fat compartment. (**a**) Schematic classification. (**b**) Cadaver superficial fat

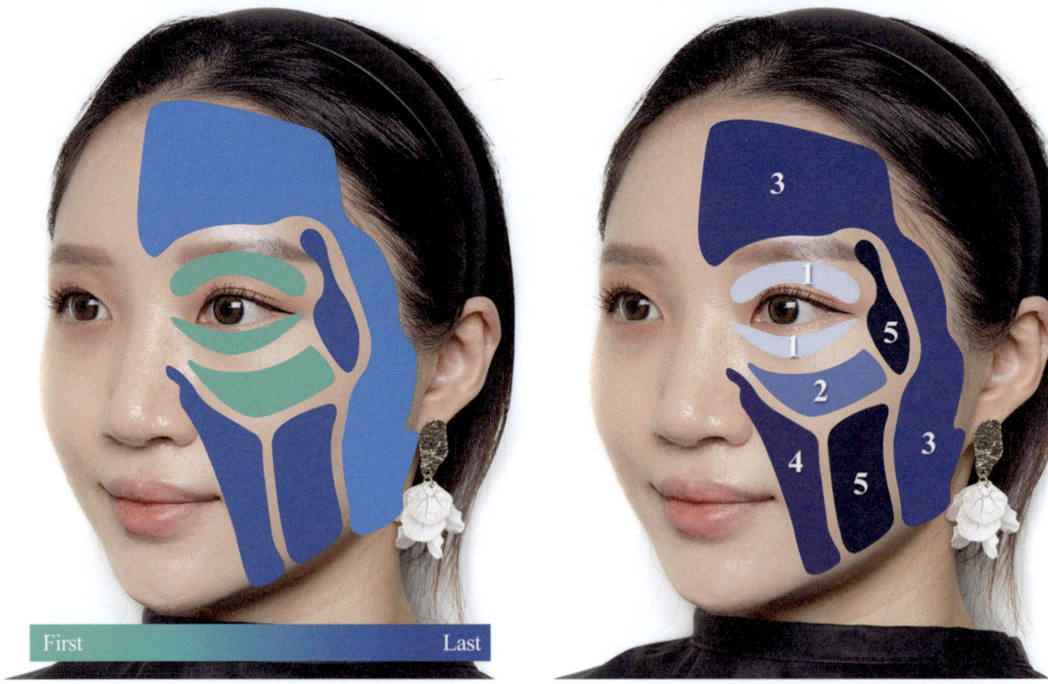
First
Last
3
1
1
5
2
3
4
5

Fig. 1.20 Changes in facial fat absorption by aging process. Periorbital (1) and malar fat pads (2) tend to be affected first in life, followed by the lateral cheek (3), deep cheek (4), and lateral temporal areas (5)

Nasolabial fat is known for its rarely deflatable nature [6]. These phenomena can help understand the aging process and should also be considered when injecting hyaluronic acid fillers.

1.5 Retaining Ligaments

There are many structures which connect the skin to bone or subcutaneous layer. Defining the facial ligaments is controversial, but these structures are important for retaining the face. Because of these structures, various grooves and furrows are formed; thus, understanding these structures is important for the hyaluronic acid filler procedure. For example, the infraorbital groove occurs due to the zygomaticocutaneous ligament, and without intervention in this ligament, correcting the groove completely using hyaluronic acid fillers becomes difficult. Thus, understanding the various ligaments can result in more precise injection (Fig. 1.21).

There are multiple structures, such as veins of the face, glands such as the parotid gland, and the facial nerve, which are not described in this chapter, as the most important structures concerning hyaluronic acid filler injection are the arteries of the face. A safer procedure can be performed by understanding the basic arterial pathway and using Doppler ultrasonography.

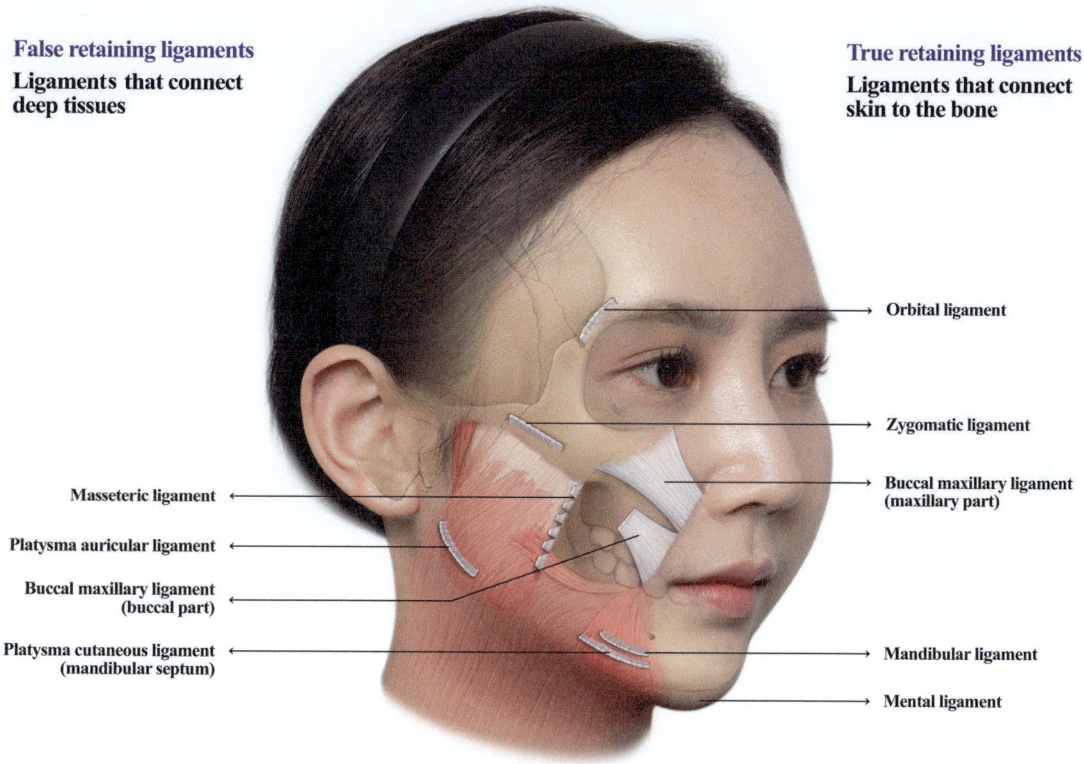

Fig. 1.21 Facial retaining ligaments

References

1. Cong LY, Phothong W, Lee SH, Wanitphakdeedecha R, Koh I, Tansatit T, Kim HJ. Topographic analysis of the supratrochlear artery and the supraorbital artery: implication for improving the safety of forehead augmentation. Plast Reconstr Surg. 2017;139(3):620e–7. https://doi.org/10.1097/PRS.0000000000003060.
2. Lee JG, Yang HM, Hu KS, Lee YI, Lee HJ, Choi YJ, Kim HJ. Frontal branch of the superficial temporal artery: anatomical study and clinical implications regarding injectable treatments. Surg Radiol Anat. 2015;37(1):61–8. https://doi.org/10.1007/s00276-014-1306-6.
3. Lee W, Moon HJ, Kim JS, Chan BL, Yang EJ. Doppler ultrasound-guided thread lifting. J Cosmet Dermatol. 2020;19(8):1921–7. https://doi.org/10.1111/jocd.13240.
4. Tansatit T, Moon HJ, Rungsawang C, Jitaree B, Uruwan S, Apinuntrum P, Phetudom T. Safe planes for injection rhinoplasty: a histological analysis of midline longitudinal sections of the Asian nose. Aesth Plast Surg. 2016;40(2):236–44. https://doi.org/10.1007/s00266-016-0621-1.
5. Lee JG, Yang HM, Choi YJ, Favero V, Kim YS, Hu KS, Kim HJ. Facial arterial depth and relationship with the facial musculature layer. Plast Reconstr Surg. 2015;135(2):437–44. https://doi.org/10.1097/PRS.0000000000000991.
6. Stuzin JM, Rohrich RJ, Dayan E. The facial fat compartments revisited: clinical relevance to subcutaneous dissection and facial deflation in face lifting. Plast Reconstr Surg. 2019;144(5):1070–8. https://doi.org/10.1097/PRS.0000000000006181.

Hyaluronic Acid Filler Properties and Rheology

2

Contents

2.1 Introduction

The hyaluronic acid filler is made by mixing hyaluronic acid (HA) with a crosslinker. HA naturally exists in the human body and is degraded by hyaluronidase. HA is mixed with a crosslinker to prevent enzymatic degradation for a longer duration. This hydrogel is formulated by various manufacturing processes, and the filler rheology can objectively reveal its properties. Rheology can be applied to all materials, from liquids to solids. Understanding filler rheology is important for estimating the longevity of the injected filler. In this chapter, we will discuss the objective parameters to understand the properties of the HA filler.

W. Lee, *Advances in Hyaluronic Acid Filler Injections*,
https://doi.org/10.1007/978-981-97-6528-7_2

2.2 Hyaluronic Acid

HA is composed of skin, joints, and vitreous bodies, and constitutes 12 g for a 70 kg human. About 3 g of HA is produced and degraded daily by the human body. HA is a disaccharide composed of glucuronic acid and glucosamine, and is a glycosaminoglycan (Fig. 2.1). HA is a polar-like substance with a high affinity for water and acts as a lubricant in the human body [1]. HA filler is gel-like structure which is composed of HA and a crosslinker, and is thus commonly known as "hydrogel." HA is evolutionarily conserved, existing in animals and bacteria, with no structural difference between the species. Thus, HA was previously extracted from rooster combs, but in recent times, *Streptococci equi zooepidemicus* is the main source [2]. Animal-based HA has been traditionally extracted from rooster combs, while non-animal-based HA is usually extracted from bacteria. Structural differences include the length of the polymer chain, the non-animal-based HA usually having 4000–6000 monomeric units and an average molecular weight of 1.5–2.5 MDa, while animal-based HA have 10,000–15,000 monomeric units and 4–6 MDa in size.

2.3 Manufacturing Process

HA filler manufacturing processes differ for each company, and the final products also differ. Products are typically distinguished from each other based on various parameters. Variations in the products arise due to parameters such as the crosslinker, temperatures, and manufacturing processes [3]. HA fillers with different properties are produced because of the different manufacturing processes.

HA powder is mixed with normal saline to form a flour-like dough. This state is called "free hyaluronic acid." When a crosslinker is added, crosslinked HA is made (Fig. 2.2). The rest of the manufacturing process is discussed in Chap. 6. Butanediol diglycidyl ether (BDDE) is commonly used as a crosslinker, while some other products contain polyethylene glycol (PEG) or divinyl sulfone (DVS). During the manufacturing process, NaOH is used to form the ether linkages of the free hydroxyl chains. Thus, ether linkages can crosslink the HA chain to other HA chains [4]. When there are more crosslinks, the cohesiveness increases, HA becomes harder, and its longevity is prolonged. Thus, when we discuss HA filler properties, we categorize them accord-

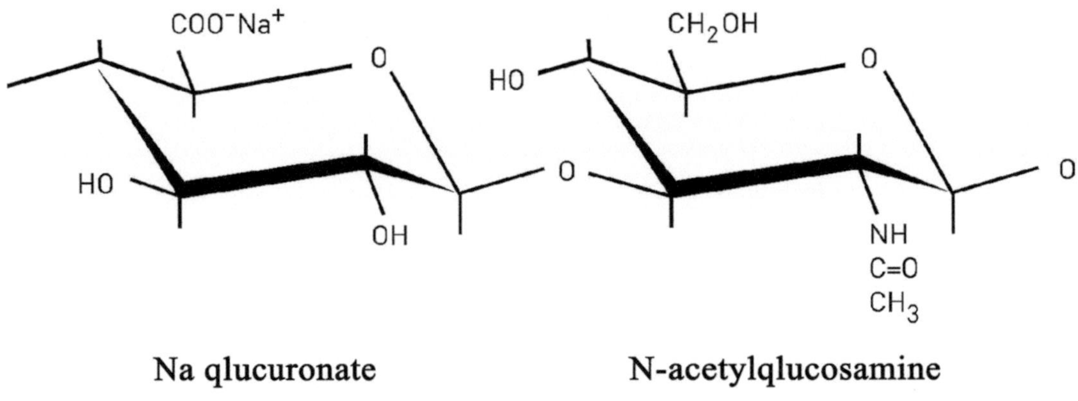

Fig. 2.1 Chemical structure of a hyaluronic acid disaccharide unit

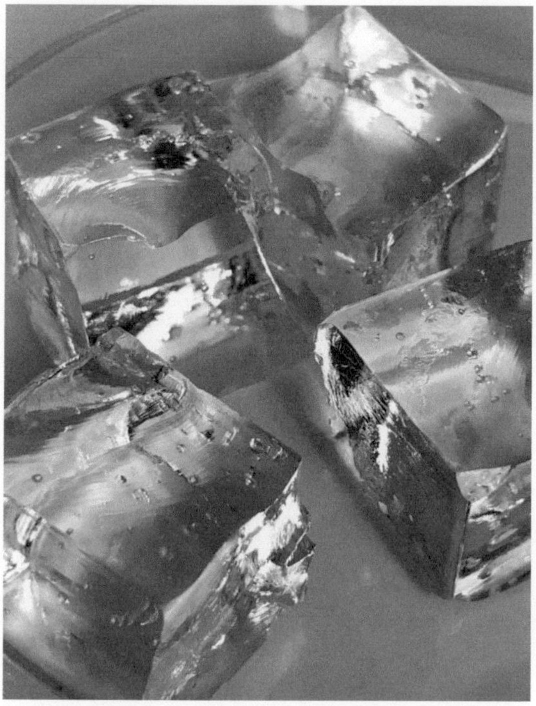

Fig. 2.2 Hyaluronic acid filler image during manufacturing process

ing to their rheology and cohesiveness. Yet, traditionally, HA fillers are classified as monophasic and biphasic fillers.

2.4 Classification by Manufacturing Process: Biphasic Versus Monophasic

After crosslinking of HA, the manufacturing process can be divided into the biphasic and monophasic end products. An example of a monophasic system is saltwater, in which different components are dissolved in one solution. An example of a biphasic system is that of ice in water which is of varying shapes but is the same component. HA filler is made with HA particles in water, and should therefore be biphasic; however, different manufacturing process usually use biphasic and monophasic processes. Biphasic fillers are distinguished from monophasic fillers by their relatively large particles and the use of a small amount of crosslinker. Thus, a small amount of crosslinker is used, and uniform particles are obtained after sieving to increase the HA gel hardness. In addition, non-cross-linked HA is used for smooth injection. By contrast, monophasic fillers tend to have relatively smoother surfaces because of the grinding process. They tend to contain a relatively large portion of the crosslinker. Monophasic fillers tend to be relatively soft but with high cohesivity. A large amount of the crosslinker can be another problem, and will be discussed in Chap. 5.

2.5 Hyaluronic Acid Filler Viscoelasticity

HA filler is a fluid-like substance with viscoelasticity. Rheology is the study of the flow of matter, primarily in the fluid state. HA filler rheology is the study of the parameters of HA filler.

2.5.1 Newtonian Fluid Versus Non-Newtonian fluid

In general, fluids can be classified as Newtonian and non-Newtonian fluids (Fig. 2.3).

A Newtonian fluid is a constant-flow fluid such as water or alcohol, and a non-Newtonian

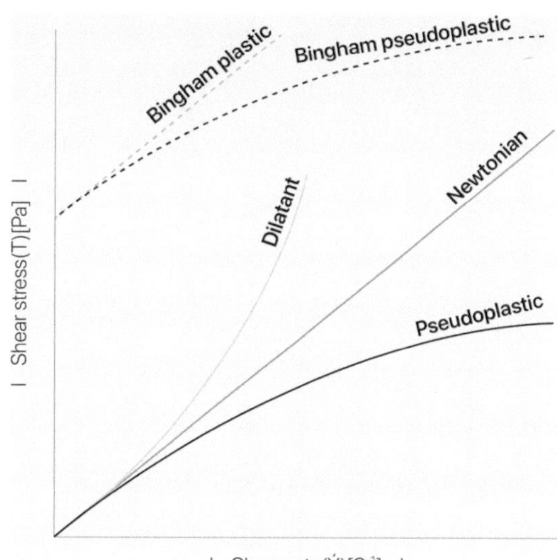

Fig. 2.3 Rheological classification of fluids

fluid is viscous like tomato ketchup or honey. Non-Newtonian fluids can be classified into dilatant and pseudoplastic fluids. The most well-known dilatant fluid is corn starch powder mixed with water. When high-power stimuli are applied to corn starch, it becomes stiffer; however, when low-power stimuli are applied, it becomes a fluid-like substance. Therefore, dilatant fluids are described as those that become more viscous when stronger stimuli are applied. On the other hand, pseudoplastic fluid is similar to tomato ketchup, which becomes a fluid-like substance after we press the tomato ketchup tube. HA filler can be compared with a pseudoplastic fluid, which is a highly viscous fluid inside a prefilled syringe, because of its low shear rate. However, when an injection force is applied and the shear rate is increased, HA filler becomes a more fluid-like substance (shear thinning) and passes through the needle. When the filler is injected into human tissue, the shear rate decreases again to become a solid-like substance (Fig. 2.4).

2.5.2 Shear Stress Versus Normal Stress

In filler rheology, external power is usually described as shear stress, as illustrated in Fig. 2.3. One of the most commonly used parameter of rheology is the elastic modulus (G′). The elastic modulus is an important parameter of fillers. The lifting capacity and longevity of the filler are associated with the elastic modulus. Elastic modulus is the parameter that defines the restoration deformation caused by shearing stress. When we press the rubber ball and remove our hand, it restores its original shape, which is an example of elastic modulus. However, when pressed by hand, the power is a compressive force and not a shearing force. Therefore, the power is the normal stress, and the elastic modulus is E′ rather than G′ (Fig. 2.5).

Shearing and normal stresses can be applied when HA filler is injected into the human face. Shearing stress constantly appears between the

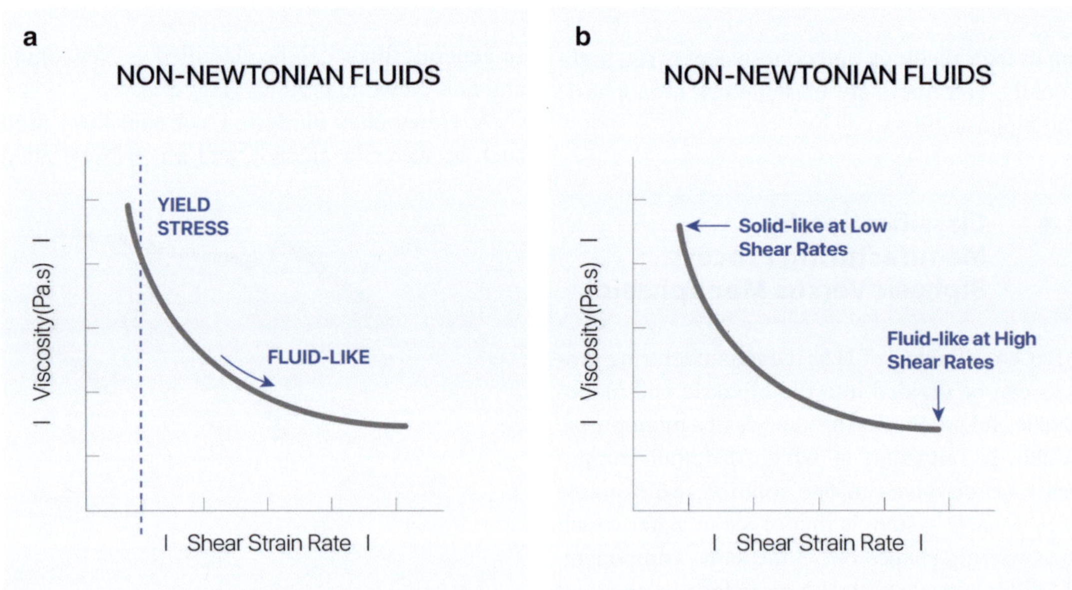

Fig. 2.4 Viscous change by shear stress rate of Hyaluronic acid filler (non newtonian fluid). (**a**) Non-newtonian fluid: yield stress. (**b**) Non newtonian fluid: solid vs fluid

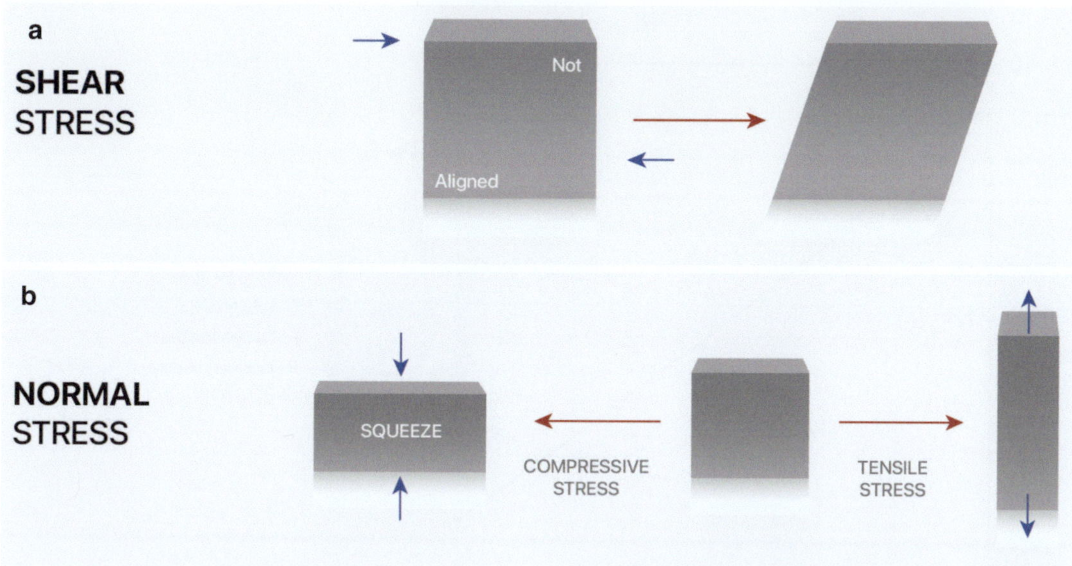

Fig. 2.5 Shearing stress (**a**) versus normal stress (**b**)

facial layers, and HA filler are meant to overcome the shearing stress so as to not deform from the original shape. However, when HA filler is injected into the nose under the nasalis muscle, a constant compressive force is applied. In addition, when HA filler is applied at the midface, a compression force can be applied because of hand compression. Therefore, not only is G′ important but E′ should also be applied while considering the rheology of the filler. Recent procedures report the injection of HA fillers in the supraperiosteal layer for vascular prevention, which yields more of a compressive force than shearing force. However, G′ is one of the most commonly used parameter of rheology, and it is important to compare the product using objective parameters.

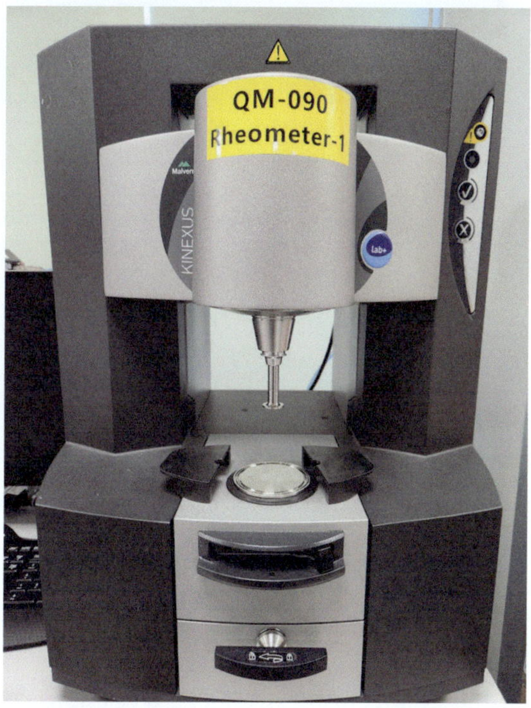

Fig. 2.6 Rheometer

2.6 Rheometer

Various rheological parameters exist, but only a few can be used when filler rheology is applied. A rheometer can be used to investigate the nature of the HA filler material to be used (Fig. 2.6).

Rheometry readings are dependent on multiple conditions, such as the plate size, temperature, and various other conditions. The frequency (Hz) of the rheometer during the analysis is especially related to the final result (Figs. 2.7 and 2.8). Thus, comparing data is more important than analyzing the parameter results alone. The

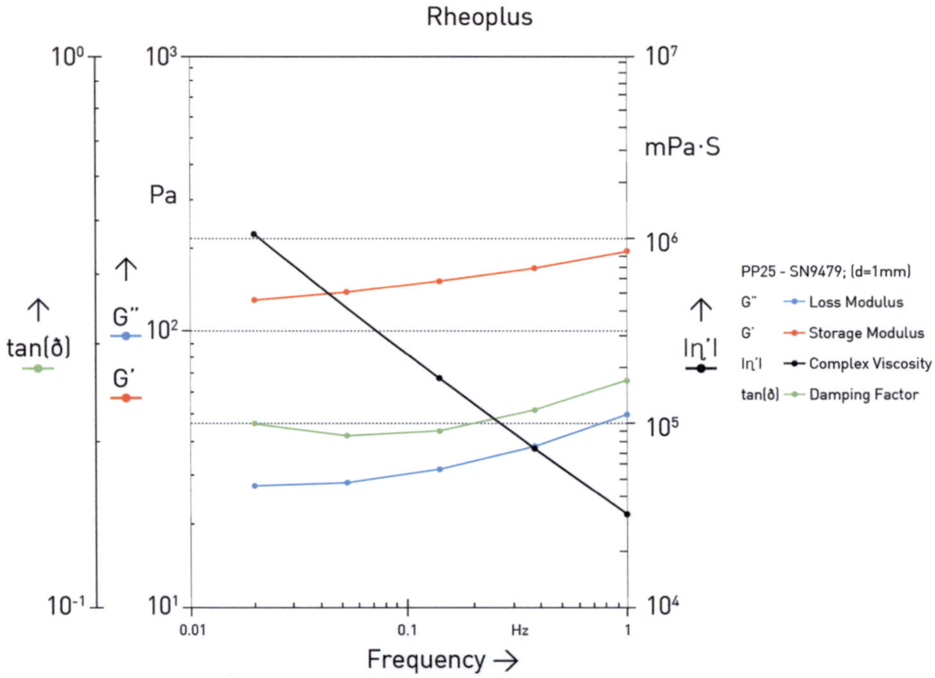

Meas. Pts.	Angular Frequency	Storage Modulus	Loss Modulus	Damping Factor	Complex Viscosity
	[rad/s]	[Pa]	[Pa]	[1]	[Pa·s]
1	6.28	1.94E+01	5.02E+01	0.258	3.19E+01
2	2.36	1.70E+02	3.89E+01	0.229	7.37E+01
3	0.889	1.52E+02	3.18E+01	0.209	1.75E+02
4	0.334	1.38E+02	2.84E+01	0.205	4.22E+02
5	0.126	1.29E+02	2.76E+01	0.214	1.05E+03

Fig. 2.7 Rheometer result of one hyaluronic acid filler; different frequency ranges

key rheometer parameters are listed in Table 2.1. In addition, the rheological parameters of 48 HA fillers (used in South Korea) are shown in Table 2.2 [5].

The property of one HA filler can be estimated upon comparison with 48 rheologic parameters, while the 48 rheologic parameters can estimate each other by tan δ or G′. For example, when tan δ is close to one, the product resembles water in clinical settings. Rheological parameters other than the injection force, particle size, and cohesiveness are discussed later.

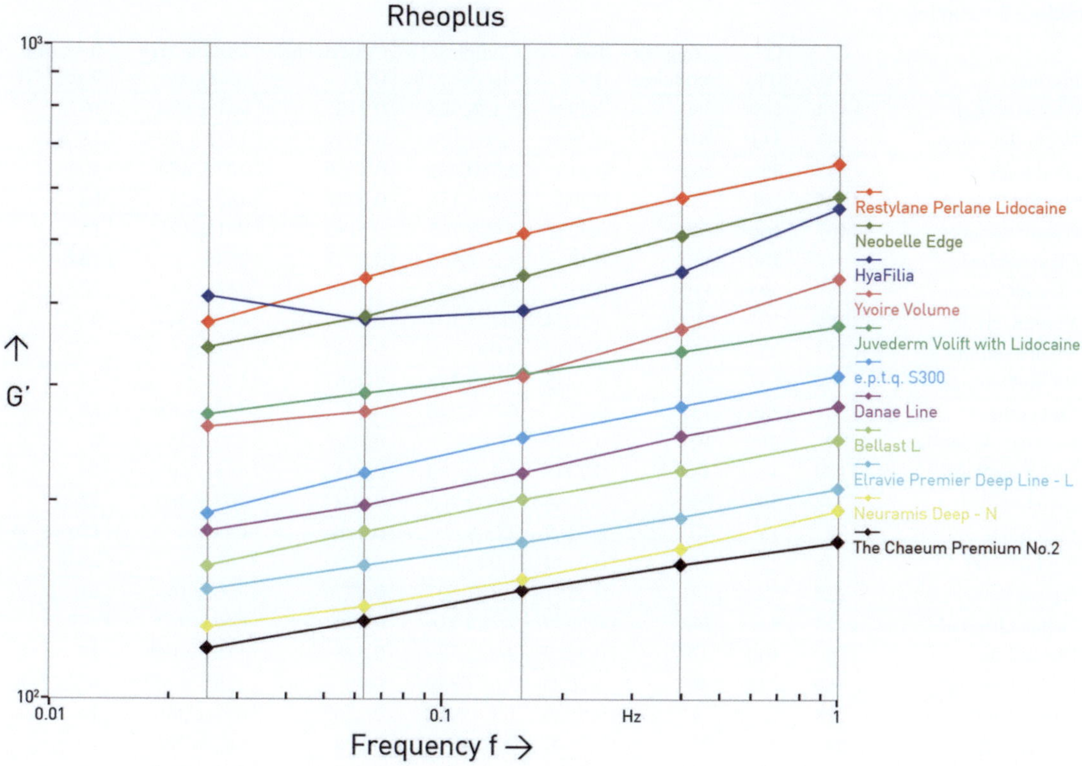

Fig. 2.8 Multiple hyaluronic acid filler G′ results by frequency

Table 2.1 Rheologic parameters relevant for hyaluronic acid filling

Terms	Definition
Elastic modulus (G′)	Energy stored and rebounded after shear stress (storage modulus)
Viscous modulus (G″)	Dissipated energy during shear stress due to friction (loss modulus)
Tan delta (Tan δ)	Division of G″ by G′ (G″/G′); measures whether a hyaluronic acid filler is more elastic or more viscous
Phase angle	This parameter involves the transformation of tan δ to an angle. When tan $\delta = 1$, then the phase angle is 90°
Complex modulus (G*)	Energy needed to deform a filler through shear stress (gel firmness or hardness). $G^* = \sqrt{(G')^2 + (G'')}\ ^2$
Complex viscosity	The parameter of a filler's ability to resist flow indicates the filler's thickness and is intimately related to the injection force

Table 2.2 Rheologic data for the hyaluronic acid products used in South Korea

Product	G′ (Pa)	G′′ (Pa)	Complex modulus	Tan delta	Complex viscosity (η)	Cohesiveness (N)	Particle size (μm/mL)	Injection force (N)
Restylane	349	145	378	0.4180	3,011,188	0.3509	547 ± 280	8
Perlane	411	199	457	0.4849	3,637,022	0.2869	1024 ± 547	16
Restylane SubQ	768	245	806	0.3190	6,420,375	0.3387	1393 ± 757	25
NeobelleSkin	372	136	396	0.3667	3,157,278	1.0296	241 ± 117	12
NeobelleBasic	365	116	383	0.3182	3,048,961	0.9481	447 ± 215	15

(continued)

Table 2.2 (continued)

Product	G′ (Pa)	G′′ (Pa)	Complex modulus	Tan delta	Complex viscosity (η)	Cohesiveness (N)	Particle size (μm/mL)	Injection force (N)
NeobelleEdge	374	110	390	0.2936	3,106,528	0.9183	941 ± 499	16
NeobelleContour	387	111	403	0.2884	3,207,126	0.9019	1472 ± 796	18
HyafiliaPetit	247	85	261	0.343	2,080,246	0.5536	227 ± 124	10
HyafiliaClassic	345	101	359	0.294	2,858,186	0.6038	488 ± 267	12
HyafiliaGrand	407	166	440	0.407	3,499,743	0.5185	991 ± 525	15
ClevielPrime	372	180	413	0.485	3,291,663	0.8778	284[a]	16.6
ClevielContour	857	694	1103	0.81	8,774,267	1.536	243[a]	20
YvoireClassic	286	103	304	0.3624	2,424,107	0.2894	693 ± 344	9.8
YvoireVolume	253	73	263	0.2910	2,097,766	0.3567	1036 ± 581	12.7
YvoireContour	484	157	509	0.3245	4,049,358	0.2867	1258 ± 742	19
CutegelMax	701	286	757	0.41	6,024,716	0.57	1106 ± 689[a]	20
JuvedermVolbella	99	21	101	0.2189	814,593	0.3046	634 ± 255	8
JuvedermVolift	179	42	184	0.2343	1,468,502	0.3417	644 ± 303	10
JuvedermVoluma	284	58	290	0.2066	2,309,805	0.4043	703 ± 389	25
E.p.t.q.S100	37	15	40	0.4269	323,859	0.4184	UD	19.6
E.p.t.q.S300	128	27	131	0.2137	1,048,864	0.6102	UD	29.4
E.p.t.q.S500	224	57	231	0.2551	1,847,607	0.8776	296 ± 168	31
Danae Original	154	81	174	0.5279	1,389,716	0.5531	646 ± 352	9.8
Danae Line	260	100	279	0.3869	2,222,574	0.3785	1162 ± 668	19
Danae Contour	469	134	488	0.2873	3,887,740	0.46	1291 ± 762	37.2
BellastVital	128	72	147	0.5636	1,170,954	0.2362	685 ± 386	15
BellastSoft L	94	22	97	0.2400	775,485	0.2285	683 ± 321	12
Bellast L	119	25	122	0.2135	969,817	0.2880	684 ± 242	16
BellastPlus	87	18	89	0.2062	714,771	0.5093	652 ± 319	32.3
BellastVolume	106	23	108	0.215	866,658	0.4458	685 ± 313	33
ElraviePremiumLight	140	34	144	0.2431	1,151,729	0.5260	UD	23
ElraviePremiumDeep line	159	39	164	0.2486	1,309,982	0.5874	UD	25
ElraviePremiumUltra volume	198	59	207	0.2985	1,646,177	0.8478	UD	24.5
Neuramis Light	4	4	6	1.0530	51,271	0.2049	322 ± 133	8
Neuramis	57	24	133	0.4284	499,532	0.4532	433 ± 178	12.7
Neuramis deep	127	38	133	0.3000	1,061,307	0.5998	411 ± 171	16.6
Neuramis volume	281	71	290	0.2551	2,309,230	0.8003	402 ± 175	22.5
Chaeum No. 1	76	28	81	0.3733	651,115	0.4888	480 ± 204	14.7
Chaeum No. 2	146	29	149	0.2036	1,193,756	0.6716	473 ± 242	34.3
Chaeum No. 3	232	52	238	0.2200	1,896,742	0.7474	596 ± 291	37.2
Chaeum No. 4	340	68	347	0.2013	2,766,277	0.9180	664 ± 348	54.8
Lorient No. 2	203	41	207	0.20	1,673,007	0.4401	UD	UD
Lorient No. 4	338	95	351	0.28	2,795,776	0.4237	UD	UD
Lorient No. 6	413	121	430	0.29	3,423,232	0.4454	UD	UD
Belotero Soft L	2.66	2.76	3.9	1.03	30,620	UD	UD	UD
Belotero Balance L	21.7	10.4	23.9	0.479	191,817	UD	UD	UD
Belotero Intense L	78	23.7	81.5	0.3040	650,018	UD	UD	UD
Belotero Volume L	168	42.5	173.3	0.2525	1,383,440	UD	UD	UD

Measured by MCR 301 rheometer (Anton Paar Co, Austria), Frequency 0.02 Hz

[a] Median, SD, standard deviation, UD, undetermined

2.7 Injection Force: Actual Power for Injecting Filler into Human

The actual power required to inject HA filler into humans is called the injection force (Fig. 2.9) [6]. As previously described, HA filler is a non-Newtonian fluid and pseudoplastic fluid, such as tomato ketchup. This means that a certain amount of power is needed to inject HA fillers into humans. Recently, several products have been developed for smooth injection with an injection force of less than 10 N (Fig. 2.10). However, the needle diameter is important in the test. When the test was performed using when the 25G needle, the injection force decreased. Therefore, injection force tests should be performed using needles of the same diameter.

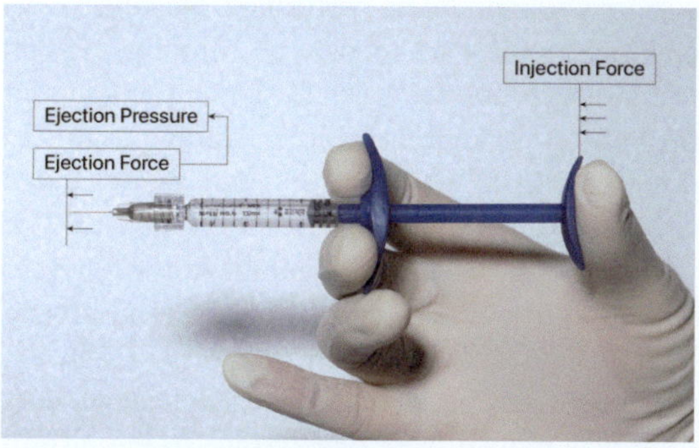

Fig. 2.9 Injection force and ejection pressure

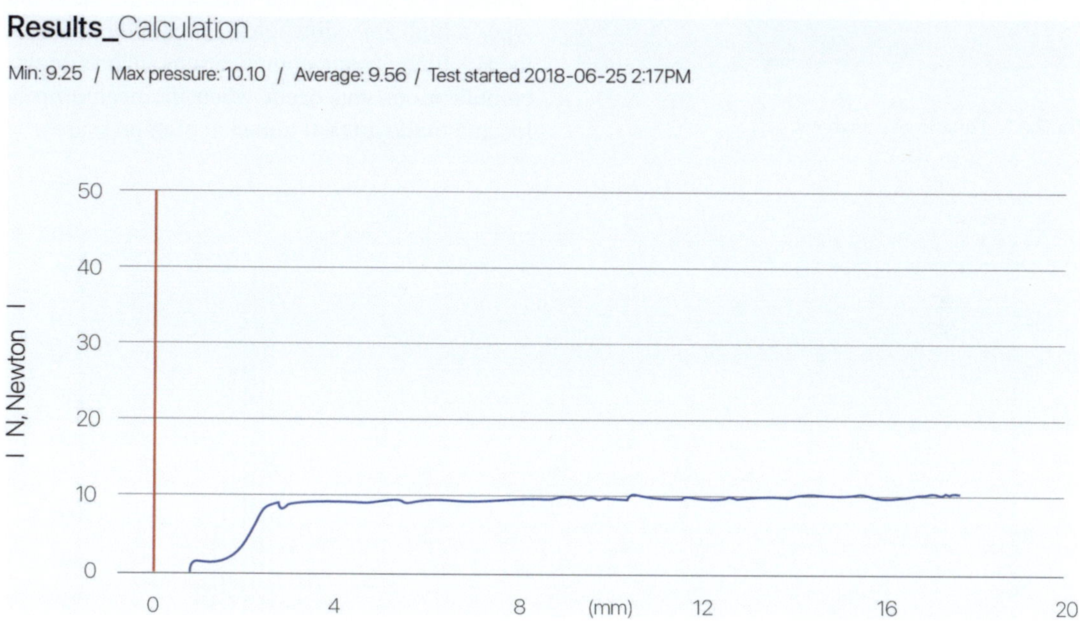

Fig. 2.10 Injection force test result

2.8 Particle Size

As described previously, the use of biphasic fillers tends to depend on the particle size. Ideally, monophasic filler particles should not be detected because of grinding; however, recently, monophasic filler particles have also been detected (Table 2.2). A particle size analyzer was used to calculate the particle size of the HA filler (Figs. 2.11 and 2.12).

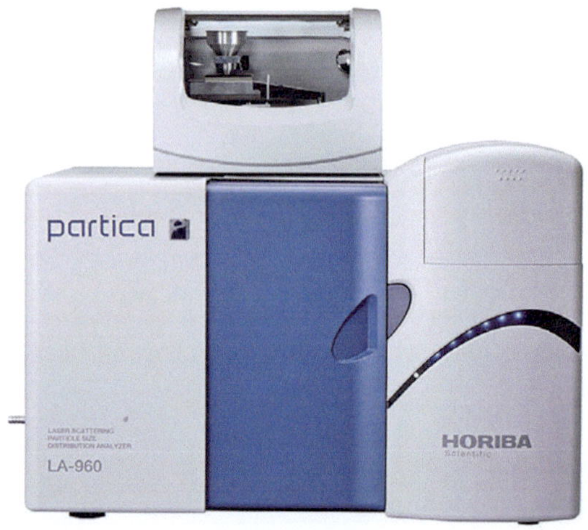

Fig. 2.11 Particle size analyzer

2.8.1 [Insulin Syringe Problems]

Some doctors use BD insulin syringes to inject HA fillers. The needle size was 30–31G so a precise injection could be performed. However, several factors must be considered before using this technique. First, the particle size can be altered by passing through the needle. A previous article described that HA rheology and particle size changed after passing 30G needle (Fig. 2.13) [7].

The second is the silicone oil in the syringe, which will be described in Chap. 6. The insulin BD syringe contained silicone oil for smooth movement of the plunge. Thus, when the HA filler was moved from one syringe to the insulin BD syringe, silicone oil was added for lubrication. The third consideration is ejection pressure. Because the syringe and needle are of the same type, a high injection force is required to inject the HA filler. Tragic complications such as ocular complications can occur when the needle tip is located in the arterial lumen at high pressure.

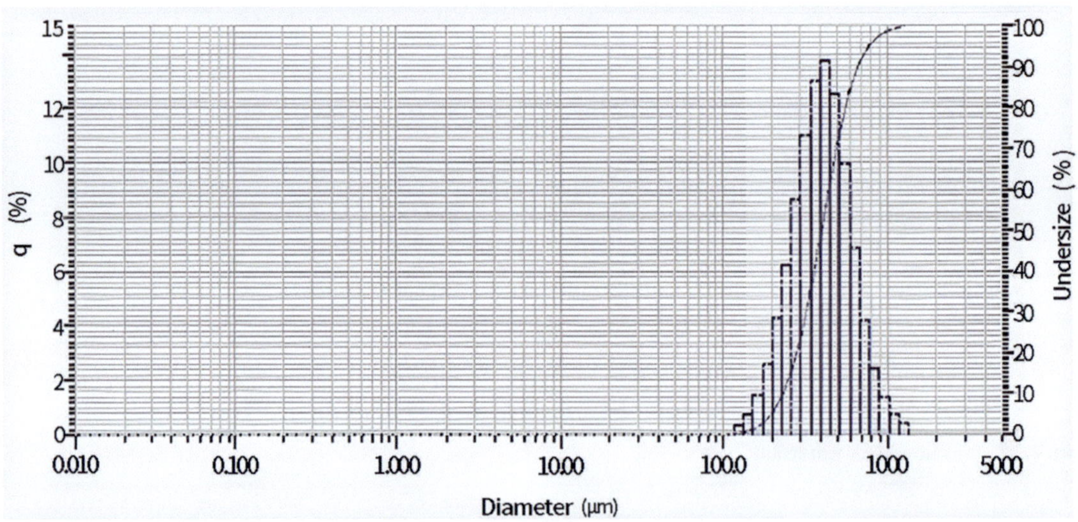

Fig. 2.12 Particle size analyzer result (average 480 µm/mL)

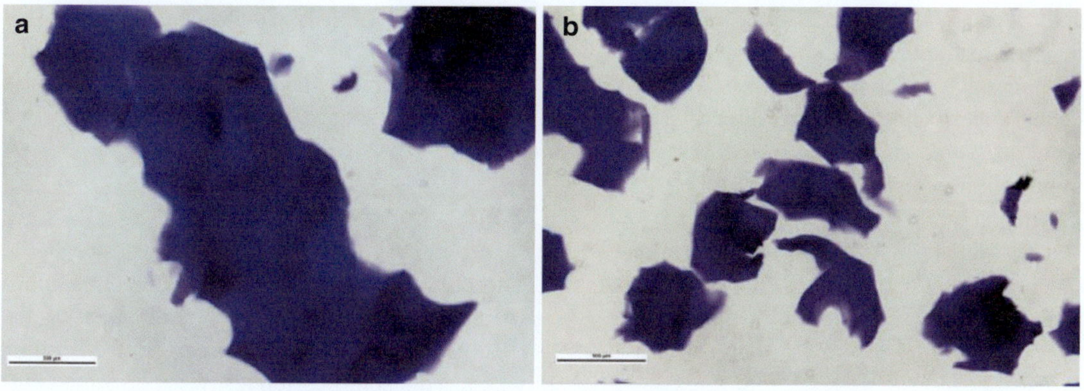

Fig. 2.13 Particle size altered after passing 30G needle. (**a**) Before. (**b**) After passing needle

Fig. 2.14 Viscosity and cohesiveness

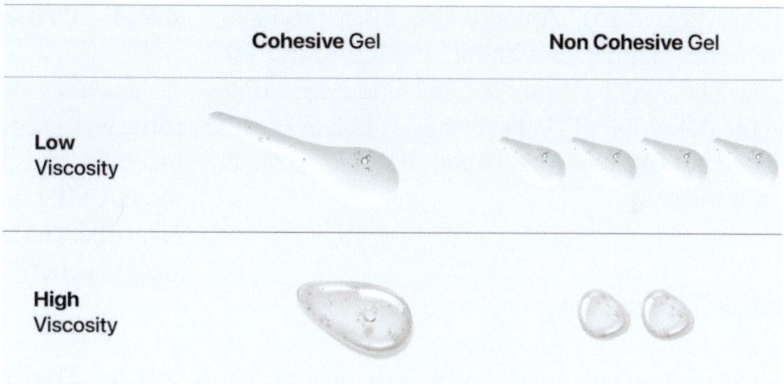

2.9 Cohesiveness

Cohesion is a link that describes the same molecular components that are attracted together. When applied to HA fillers, cohesion is the force that holds HA molecules together. Adhesion is a term by which different components adhere together. One of the best examples is mercury, which can stick together with other mercury molecules but not with other molecules. Mercury is highly cohesive but not adhesive. In the field of plastic surgery, breast implants made of silicone (cohesive gel implants) are highly cohesive and adhesive. Thus, cohesion can be distinguished from adhesion.

Cohesion of the HA filler means that the HA molecules stick together. More specifically, the cohesion of the HA filler is a molecular bond between the carboxyl chain of HA and the hydroxyl chains of other HA molecules. However, as described earlier, HA fillers contain a crosslinker. The amount of crosslinker affected the cohesiveness of the HA product. The crosslinker also affected the adhesiveness of the HA product.

Adhesion is associated with the HA filler viscosity. High-viscosity HA fillers tend to adhere to the needle lumen when injected. Thus, it is important to understand the relationship between the cohesion and viscosity (Fig. 2.14).

As previously described, when external forces such as shear stress and/or compression stress develop, the HA filler tends to be viscous, and when the stress disappears, it should be cohesive enough to maintain the shape. Therefore, cohesion is important for HA fillers. Even if the elastic modulus is high, high stress can excel at the threshold and cause irreversible deformation. Therefore, it is important to maintain the initial shape using cohesiveness. Therefore, HA filler cohesiveness affects the lifting capacity rather than the maintenance of shape.

Generally, monophasic fillers tend to exhibit better cohesiveness and are directly associated with crosslinkers. Proper crosslinking is very important for cohesiveness, and will be discussed in Chap. 5.

Unfortunately, it has not been developed for objective assessment of HA filler cohesiveness. Various tests were proposed for this purpose [8].

2.9.1 Cohesion Perceived Test

The basic test was performed using a human hand (Fig. 2.15). Among HA filler products, some can aggregate without sticking to the fingers. This may be the most reliable test according to the definition of "cohesiveness"; however, this test is not objective and cannot be used in medical science.

2.9.2 Tack Test

A tack test was performed using a rheometer. The rheometer parameters were calculated using the shearing force. However, the tack test was performed when the rheometer plate was pulled upward (Fig. 2.16). The cohesiveness results that are shown in Table 2.2 were calculated using the tack test. Thus, the tack test not only calculates cohesiveness but also includes adhesiveness.

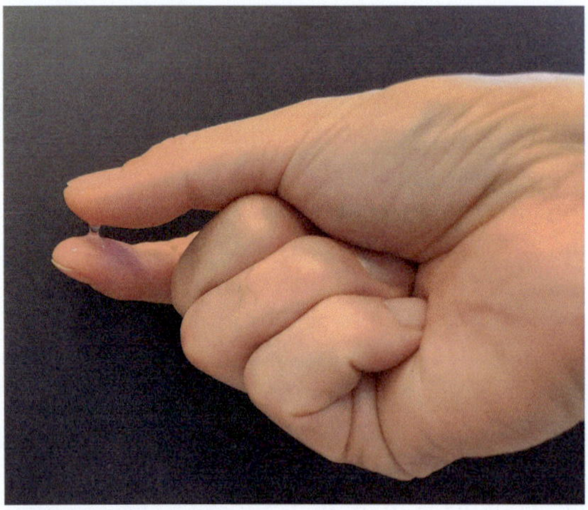

Fig. 2.15 Perceived cohesion test

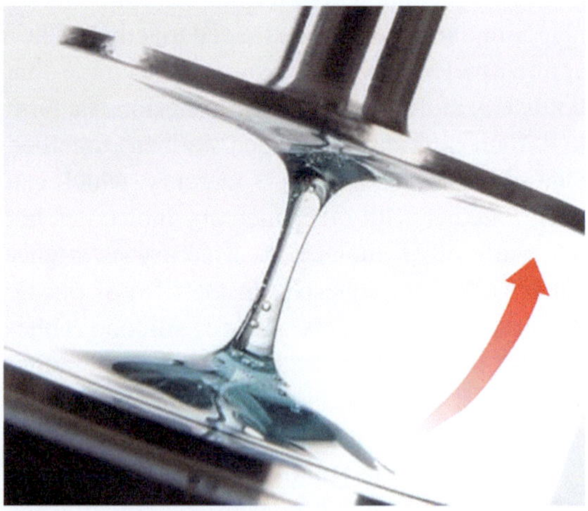

Fig. 2.16 Tack test (Rheometer)

2.9.3 Compression Test

The compression tests were performed using a rheometer. The viscoelastic parameters of the rheometer were calculated during plate shearing, whereas the compression test was performed during plate compression.

2.9.4 Drop Weight Test

A machine that typically calculates injection force was used for the drop weight test. When the machine, constantly pushes the HA filler syringe, the HA filler drops fall, weighing 20 drops. If the HA filler is highly cohesive, the decrease in weight is large.

2.9.5 Dispersion Time Test

The blue-dyed HA filler was then poured into a water tank and stirred at a constant rate. A magnetic stir bar (25 mm in length) was used at a constant rate of 170 rpm. Dispersion was evaluated using serial photographs. Each photograph was evaluated on a scale of fully dispersed, partially dispersed, partially cohesive, and fully cohesive (Fig. 2.17).

The rheological test results were compared with those of multiple cohesion tests (Fig. 2.18). As previously discussed, not all tests accurately define the cohesiveness of HA fillers. In addition, there is no consensus on the extent to which cohesion requires an ideal HA filler. This indicates that, if the cohesion is too low, the HA filler can disperse and migrate. However, if the cohesion is too high, the HA filler can aggregate in one specific area because of facial muscle movement. A large bolus of the filler can be recognized as a foreign body by the immune system.

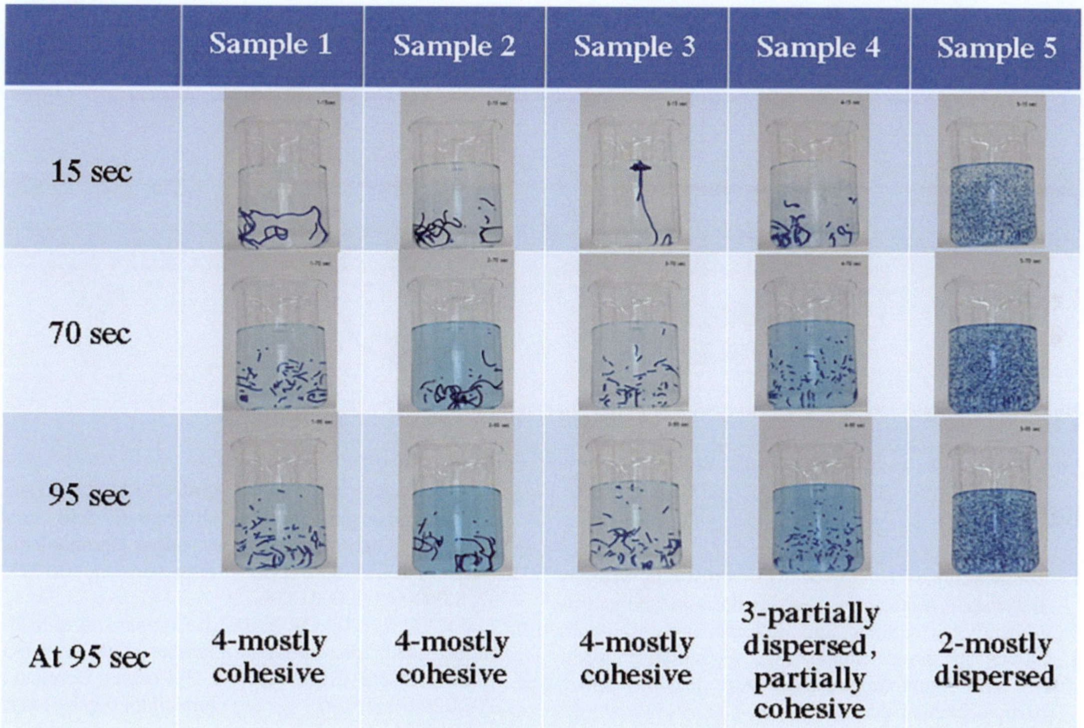

Fig. 2.17 Dispersion time test (5 HA fillers were analyzed)

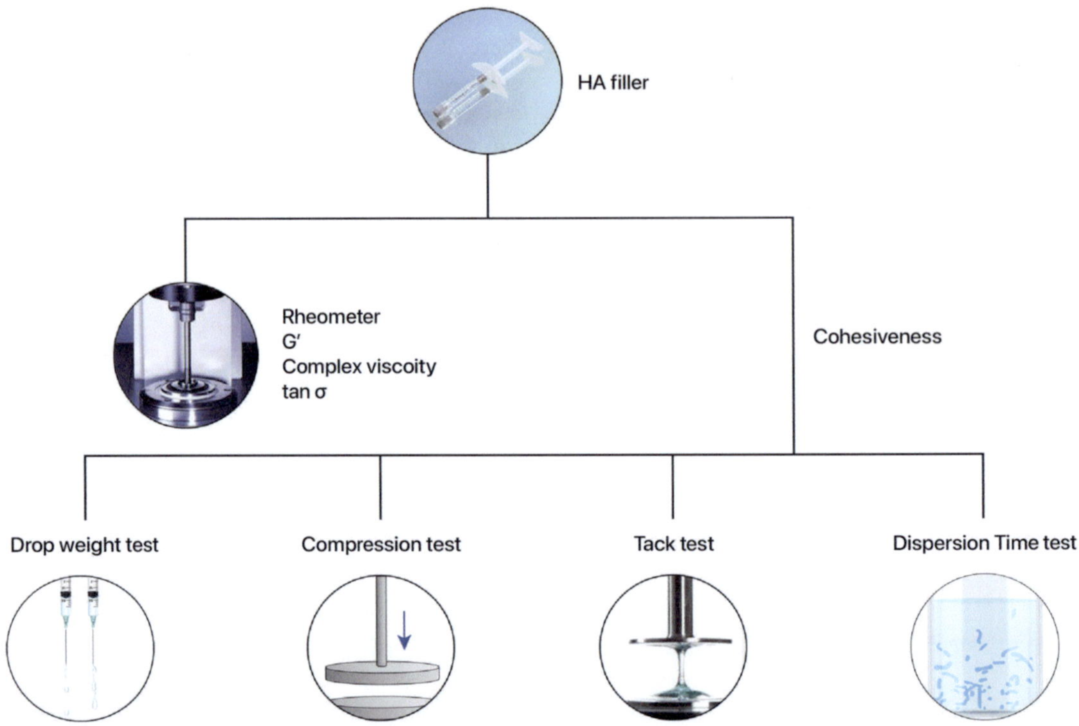

Fig. 2.18 Multiple cohesion tests compared with rheological result

References

1. Knopf-Marques H, Pravda M, Wolfova L, Velebny V, Schaaf P, Vrana NE, et al. Hyaluronic acid and its derivatives in coating and delivery systems: applications in tissue engineering, regenerative medicine and immunomodulation. Adv Healthc Mater. 2016;5(22):2841–55.
2. Mei JF, Dong ZH, Yi Y, Zhang YL, Ying GQ. A simple method for the production of low molecular weight hyaluronan by in situ degradation in fermentation broth. E-Polymers. 2019;19(1):477–81.
3. Micheels P, Sarazin D, Tran C, Salomon D. Effect of different crosslinking technologies on hyaluronic acid behavior: a visual and microscopic study of seven hyaluronic acid gels. J Drugs Dermatol. 2016;15(5):600–6.
4. Schante CE, Zuber G, Herlin C, Vandamme TF. Chemical modifications of hyaluronic acid for the synthesis of derivatives for a broad range of biomedical applications. Carbohyd Polym. 2011;85(3):469–89.
5. Lee W, Hwang SG, Oh W, Kim CY, Lee JL, Yang EJ. Practical guidelines for hyaluronic acid soft-tissue filler use in facial rejuvenation. Dermatologic Surg. 2020;46(1):41–9. https://doi.org/10.1097/DSS.0000000000001858.
6. Lee Y, Oh SM, Lee W, Yang EJ. Comparison of hyaluronic acid filler ejection pressure with injection force for safe filler injection. J Cosmet Dermatol. 2021;20(5):1551–6. https://doi.org/10.1111/jocd.14064.
7. Lee W, Oh W, Moon HJ, Koh IS, Yang EJ. Soft tissue filler properties can be altered by a small-diameter needle. Dermatologic Surg. 2020;46(9):1155–62. https://doi.org/10.1097/DSS.0000000000002220.
8. Edsman KLM, Öhrlund Å. Cohesion of hyaluronic acid fillers: correlation between cohesion and other physicochemical properties. Dermatologic Surg. 2018;44(4):557–62. https://doi.org/10.1097/DSS.0000000000001370.

3 Ultrasound Guided Hyaluronic Acid Filler Injection: Internal Carotid Artery Territories

Contents

3.1 Introduction

After having knowledge of basic anatomy of arteries of the face, it is recommended to perform Doppler ultrasound detection for more prevention of vascular complication. Learning curve is needed to perform ultrasound, but once you learn using ultrasound, safer hyaluronic acid (HA) filler injection can be performed. In this chapter, we will describe how to perform ultrasound guided HA filler injection at internal carotid artery territories. A relatively safer technique is needed at internal carotid artery territories because of a serious complication, which is ocular complication [1, 2].

3.2 Ultrasound Wave Frequency

8–17 MHz frequency can cover all layers of the face. Generally 8 MHz can detect 50 mm depth and 20 MHz can detect 10 mm depth (Fig. 3.1). Doppler ultrasound can detect both artery and vein. Artery and vein can show both red and blue color depending on blood flow, thus artery is not always red color. Method to distinguish whether

W. Lee, *Advances in Hyaluronic Acid Filler Injections*,
https://doi.org/10.1007/978-981-97-6528-7_3

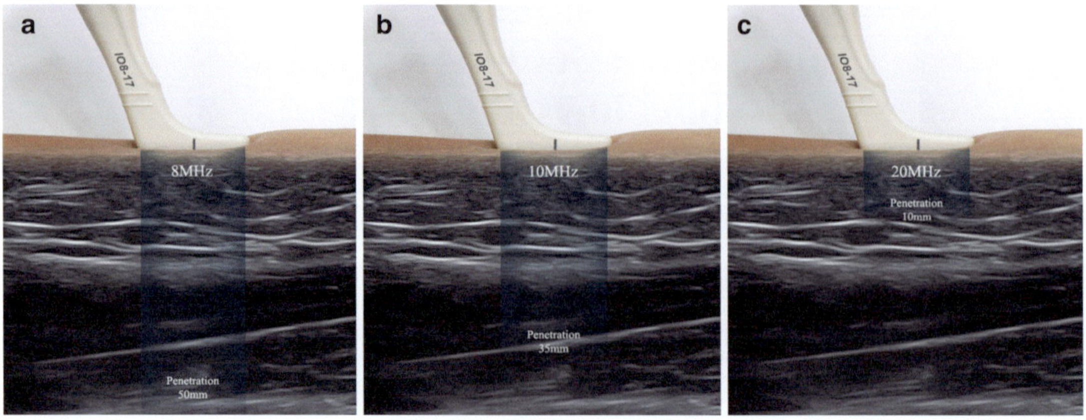

Fig. 3.1 Different depths of visualization with different frequencies: (**a**) 8 MHz (**b**) 10 MHz, and (**c**) 20 MHz

it is artery or vein is not the color but pressure of the probe. The artery does not disappear when probe pressure is applied [3].

3.3 Glabellar Wrinkle Correction

Glabellar wrinkle is made because of repetitive movement of corrugator supercilii muscle, thus usually botulinum toxin is needed to correct glabellar frown wrinkle. But repetitive wrinkle formation can develop to deeper furrow, and sometimes HA filler is needed to correct furrow. To correct glabellar wrinkle, it is recommended to inject superficially, such as dermal layer of subdermal layer [4]. When HA filler is injected into the deeper, subcutaneous layer, larger amount of HA filler is needed and it is relatively difficult to perform more precise correction (Fig. 3.2). When Doppler ultrasound is perform at glabellar wrinkle sometimes supratrochlear artery is detected (Fig. 3.3). The detected supratrochlear artery tends to run superficially, which is subdermal layer (Fig. 3.4); and sometimes it tends to run deeply, which is subcutaneous layer (Fig. 3.5).

As described previously, HA filler is recommended to inject at subdermal layer, but as seen in the Doppler ultrasound image, supratrochlear artery can be located at subdermal layer. When needle tip is located at the supratrochlear artery, ocular complication can occur. Therefore it is recommended to use Doppler ultrasound before glabellar wrinkle correction. Among the different HA fillers, author uses Lorient No. 2 or No. 4 based on rheology (Table 3.1) [5]. It is recommended to compress ophthalmic artery pathway during HA filler injection even if after detecting supratrochlear artery by Doppler ultrasound (Fig. 3.6) [6].

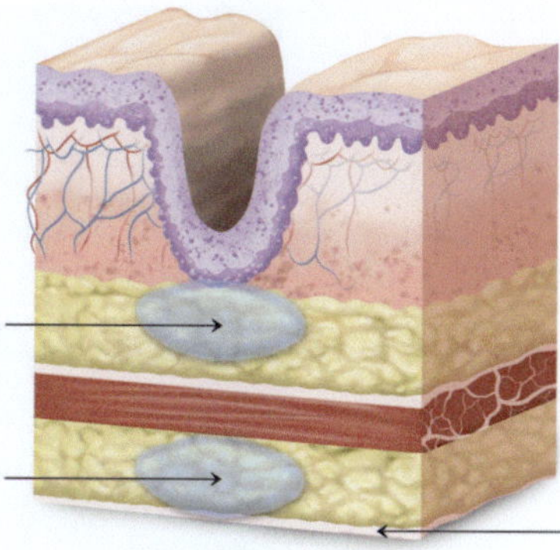

Fig. 3.2 HA filler injection layer to correct glabellar wrinkle (dermis or subdermis: more accurate wrinkle correction; submuscular layer: large amount of HA filler is needed)

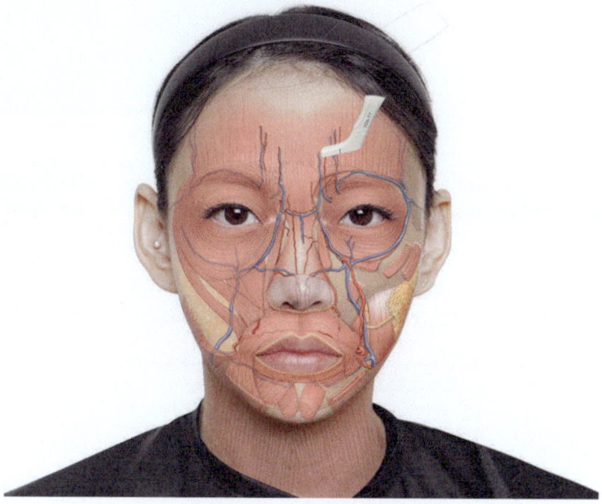

Fig. 3.3 Doppler ultrasound probe and supratrochlear artery

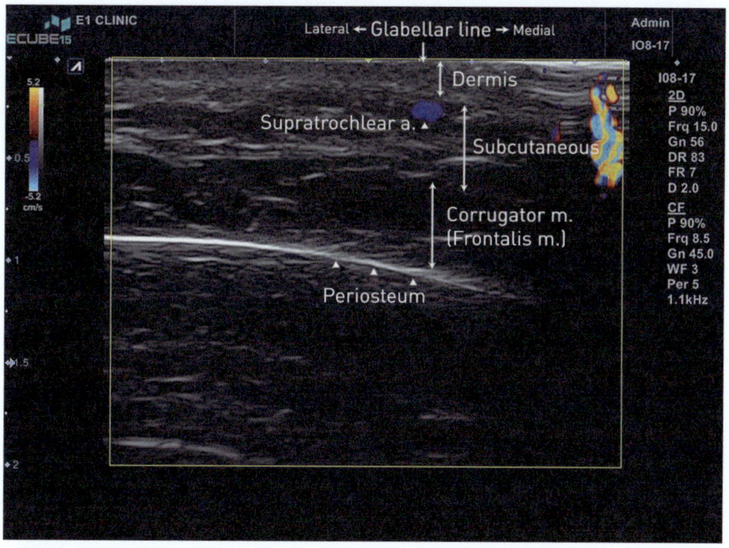

Fig. 3.4 Supratrochlear artery located at glabellar wrinkle at subdermis layer

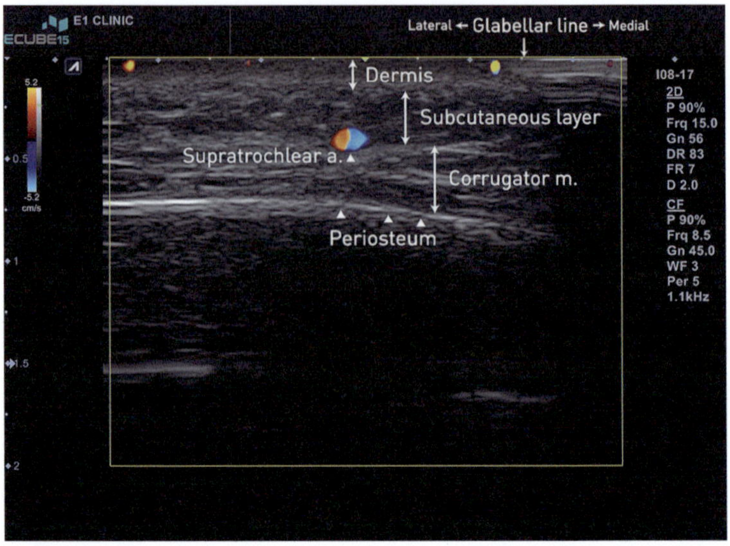

Fig. 3.5 Supratrochlear artery located at deep subcutaneous layer

Table 3.1 Hyaluronic acid fillers rheologic data [(Frequency 0.02 Hz) MCR 301 rheometer (Anton Paar Co. Austria)]

Product	G′ (Pa)	G″ (Pa)	Complex viscosity (μ)	Tan delta	Cohesiveness (N)
Lorient No. 2	203	41	1,673,007	0.20	0.4401
Lorient No. 4	338	95	2,795,776	0.28	0.4237
Lorient No. 6	413	121	3,423,232	0.29	0.4454

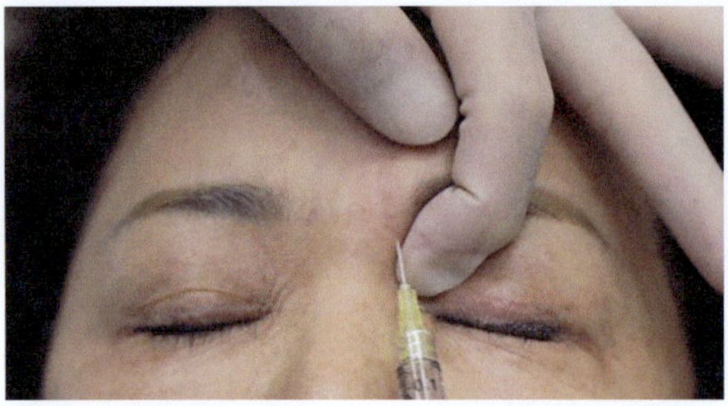

Fig. 3.6 HA filler injection by compression at ophthalmic artery branch pathway

3.4 Forehead Augmentation

Forehead is a relatively wide area and one of the most important thing for forehead augmentation by HA filler injection is not to cause irregularity. One of the important considerations of forehead augmentation is to decide the most protruded location of forehead and the supraorbital ridge. So it is important to estimate skull shape and muscle location (Fig. 3.7). It is recommended to inject under frontalis muscle so as to not cause irregularity and also because of arterial location.

Arteries of forehead area are supratrochlear artery, supraorbital artery, and frontal branch of superficial temporal artery. These three arteries can be detected using Doppler ultrasound (Figs. 3.8 and 3.9).

After vascular mapping, it is recommended to make puncture near eyebrow area and inject HA filler (Fig. 3.10). When injecting HA filler in the medial portion of forehead, one should be careful of supratrochlear deep branch and when injecting HA filler in the lateral portion of forehead, one should be careful of sentinel vein [7]. Usually submuscular layer injection is recommended because of vascular complication and also not to cause irregularity (Fig. 3.11) [8]. One consideration is the repetitive movement of frontalis muscle can make injected HA filler to be aggregated. The shape of forehead is most important, and therefore before finishing the injection, it is recommended to make patient sit in upright position and inject HA filler finally observing the forehead shape (Fig. 3.12). Lorient No. 4 is recommended based on rheology (Table 3.1).

3.4.1 Pre- and Postoperative Photograph (Figs. 3.13 and 3.14)

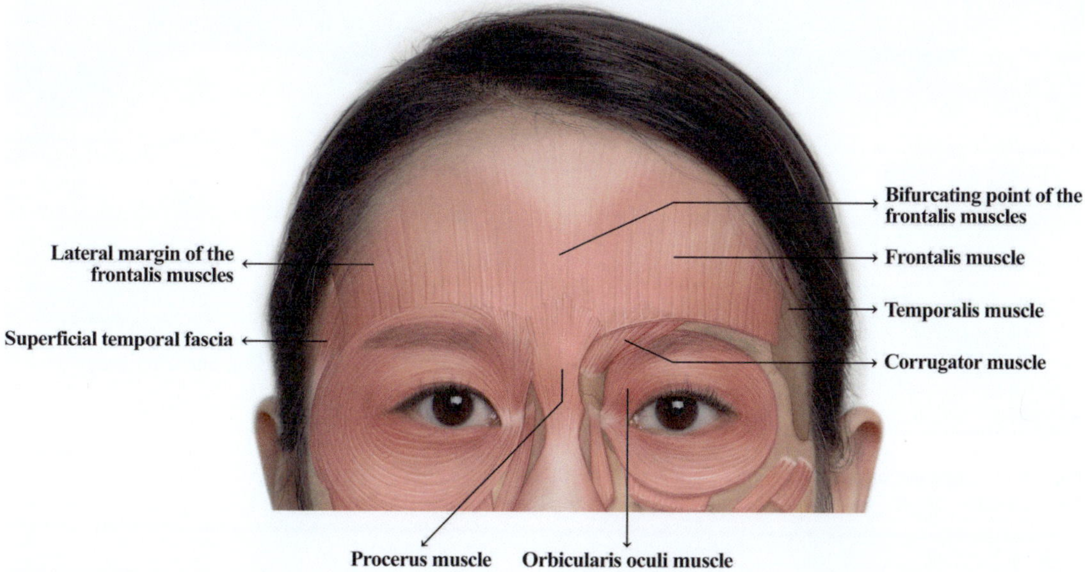

Fig. 3.7 Consideration of forehead augmentation. Frontalis muscle tends to be located lateral to superficial temporal fascia

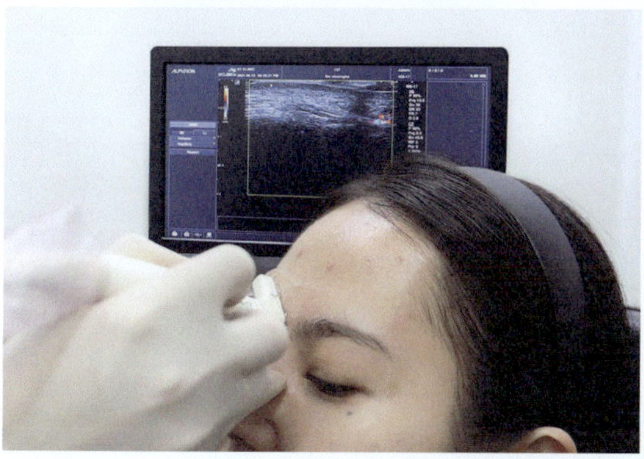

Fig. 3.8 Doppler ultrasound detection before forehead augmentation

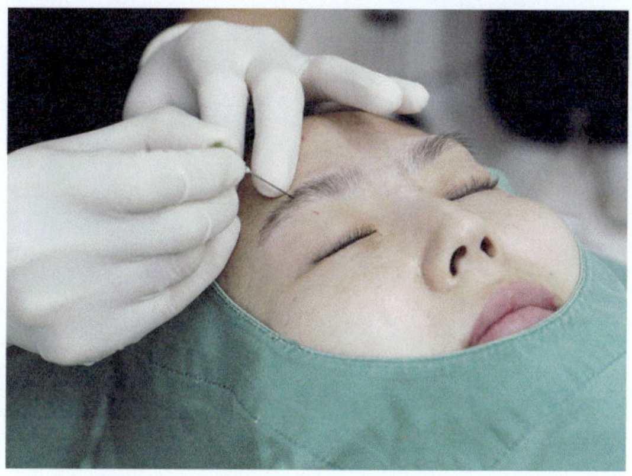

Fig. 3.10 Puncture at upper eyebrow area

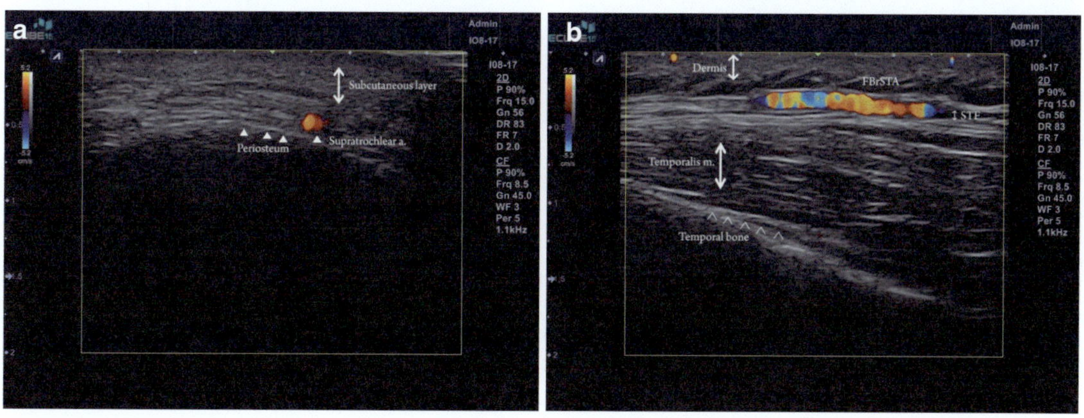

Fig. 3.9 Arteries of forehead area. (**a**) Supratrochlear artery. (**b**) Frontal branch of superficial temporal artery

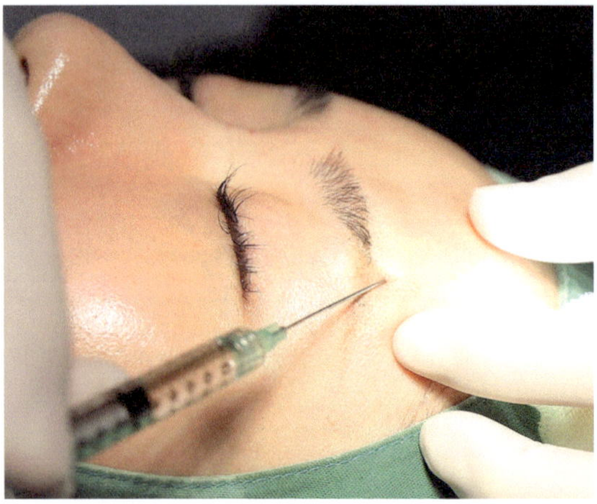

Fig. 3.11 Supraperiosteal layer gentle injection with 19G cannula

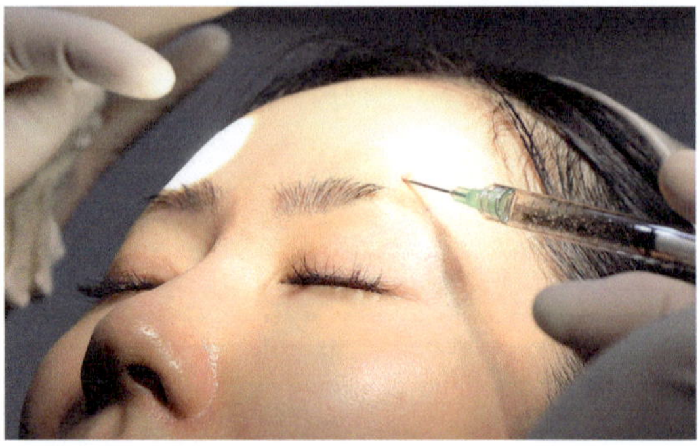

Fig. 3.12 Finish operation with checking irregularity at upright position

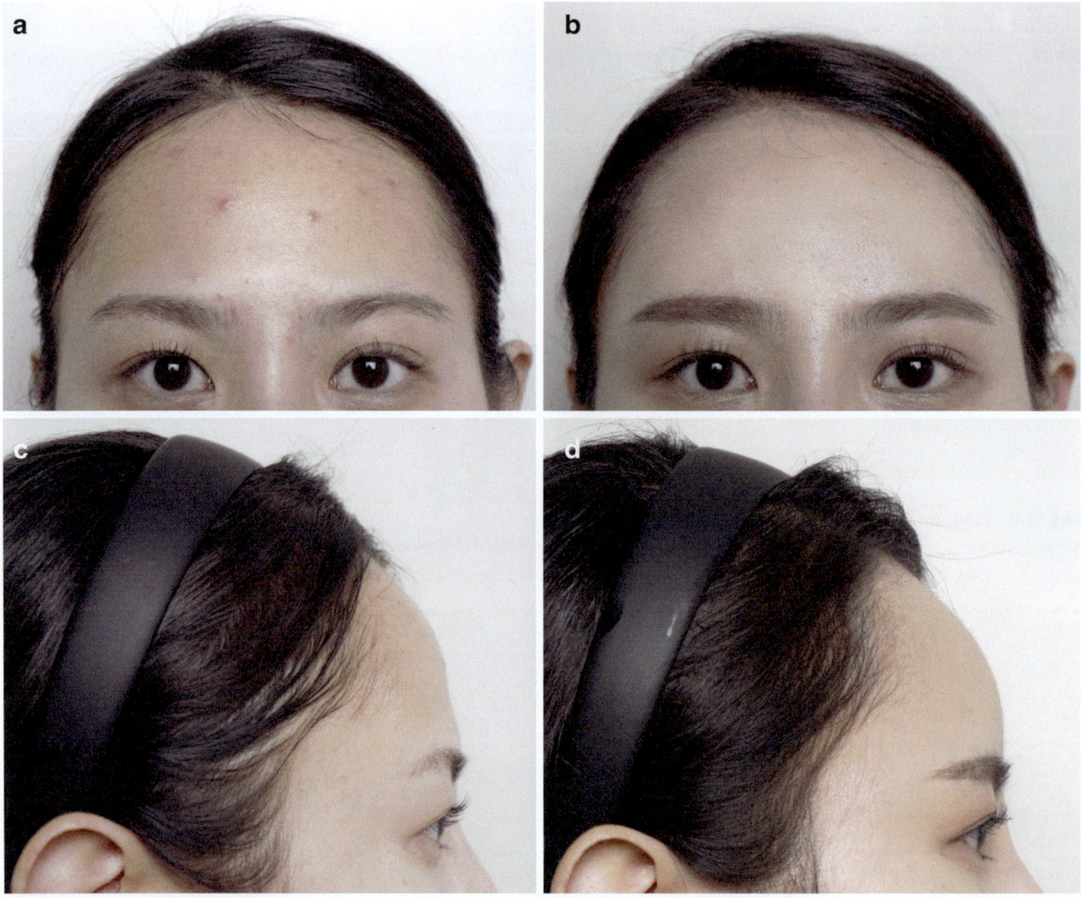

Fig. 3.13 Injection of hyaluronic acid filler in a 23-year-old woman. (**a**) Preoperative frontal view. (**b**) Postoperative frontal view after 2 weeks. (**c**) Preoperative lateral view. (**d**) Postoperative lateral view after 2 weeks

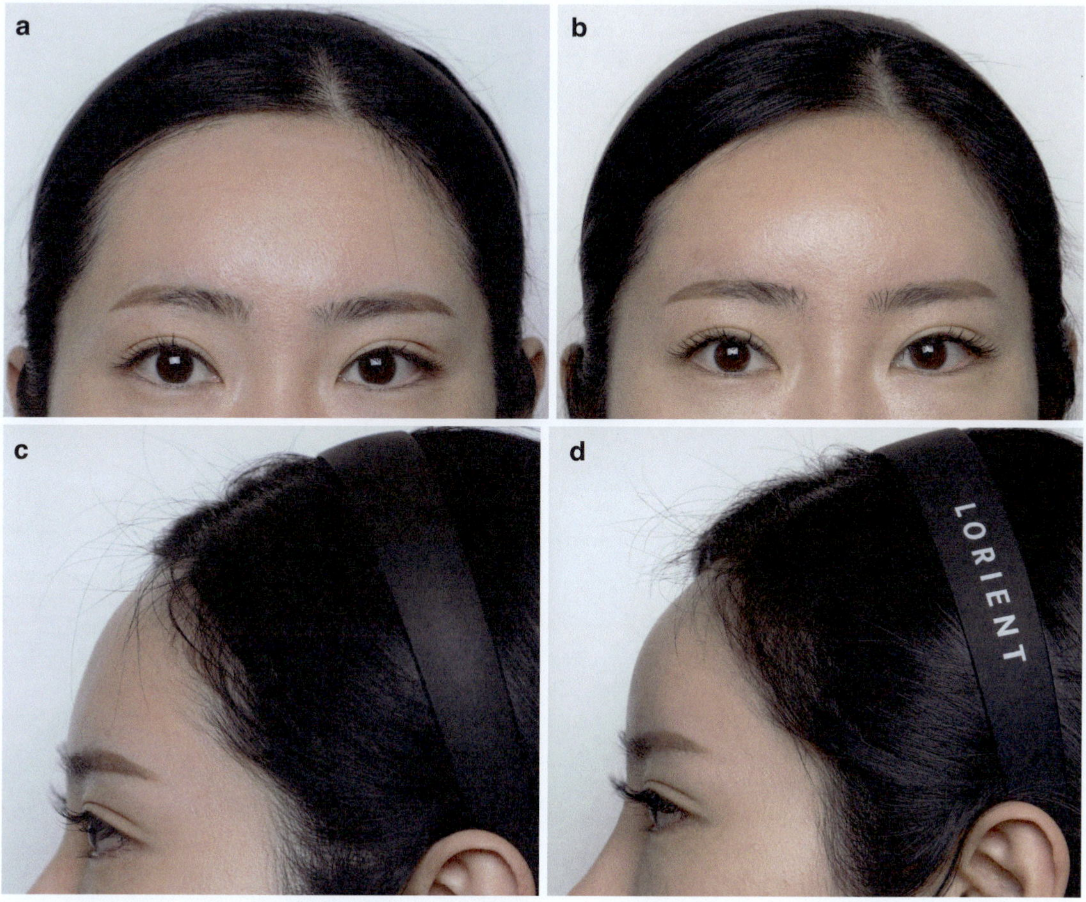

Fig. 3.14 Injection of hyaluronic acid filler in a 36-year-old woman. (**a**) Preoperative frontal view. (**b**) Postoperative frontal view after 2 weeks. (**c**) Preoperative lateral view. (**d**) Postoperative lateral view after 2 weeks

3.5 Nose Augmentation

Nose augmentation by HA filler is the easiest method to augment nose. But it is the highest incidence area of ocular complication induced by HA filler [6]. It is the most dangerous area of HA filler injection because dorsal nasal artery which supplies dorsum of nose is a branch of the ophthalmic artery. So when injecting HA filler into dorsum of nose, the layer should be decided, that is whether the injection layer will be deeper than muscle or subdermal layer because nasal vasculature tend to run at subcutaneous layer. Usually it is recommended to inject at supraperiosteal layer, but sometimes vasculature appears at deep area [8]. When injecting into deep portion, HA filler can be dispersed and wide looking appearance could be found because HA filler is viscoelastic material and deep area is constantly affected by compression force.

Nose vasculature can be detected by Doppler ultrasound before HA filler injection (Fig. 3.15). Dorsal nasal artery tends to cross midline of nose, so it is recommended to detect the artery by Doppler ultrasound and detour injecting HA filler at nose.

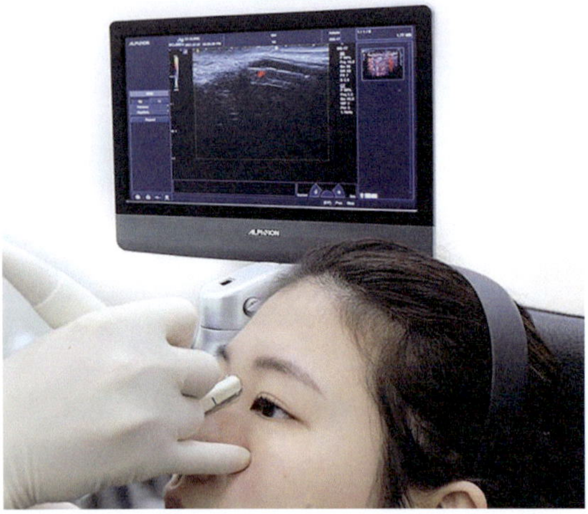

Fig. 3.15 Doppler ultrasound detection at nose

3.5.1 Nose Injection Technique by Blunt Cannula

Nose dorsum augmentation technique using cannula from infralobular entry point (Fig. 3.16). Cannula tip should be located at supraperiosteal layer. One should not be 100% confident using cannula because there is case report of ocular complication using 25G cannula [9]. Thus, it is safer to use bigger diameter blunt cannula and should feel that cannula tip is located at supraperiosteal layer.

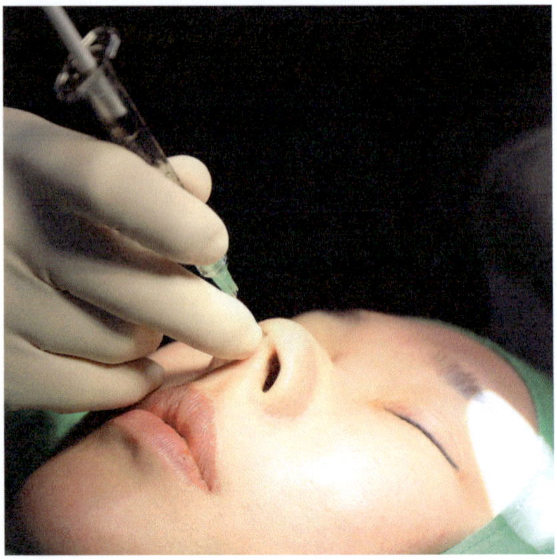

Fig. 3.16 Infralobular approach using blunt cannula. When cannular tip meets nasal bone, it is important to scratch nasal bone to locate cannula tip at supraperiosteal layer

3.5.2 Nose Injection Technique Using Sharp Needle

Needle injection is better for precise injection of HA filler. But since needle end is sharp, the possibility of vascular compromise increases. Even after Doppler ultrasound detection, it is recommended to compress lateral side of nose, which is a potent pathway of ophthalmic artery (Fig. 3.17).

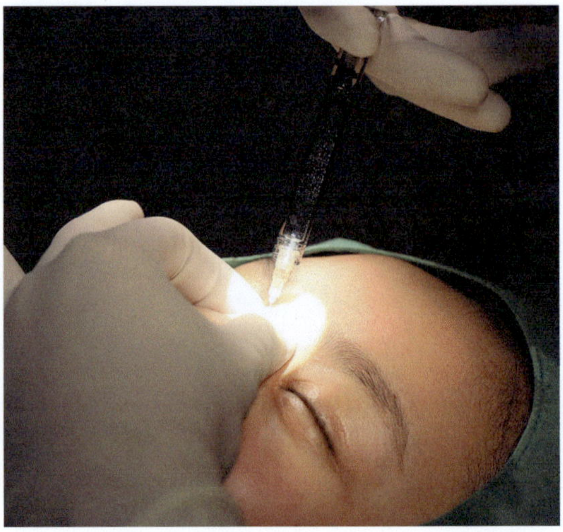

Fig. 3.17 Direct perpendicular HA filler injection at nose. Needle tip should be located at supraperiosteal layer

3.5.3 Widening Nose

Wide looking dorsum of nose area appears when constant compression force by nasalis muscle develops. Thus when injecting HA filler at nose or chin area, it is recommended to use high G′ HA filler (Table 3.1). When dorsum of the nose looks widened, it is recommended to remove first and inject HA filler again. Previous literature describes that injected hyaluronidase for degraded HA filler would disappear completely

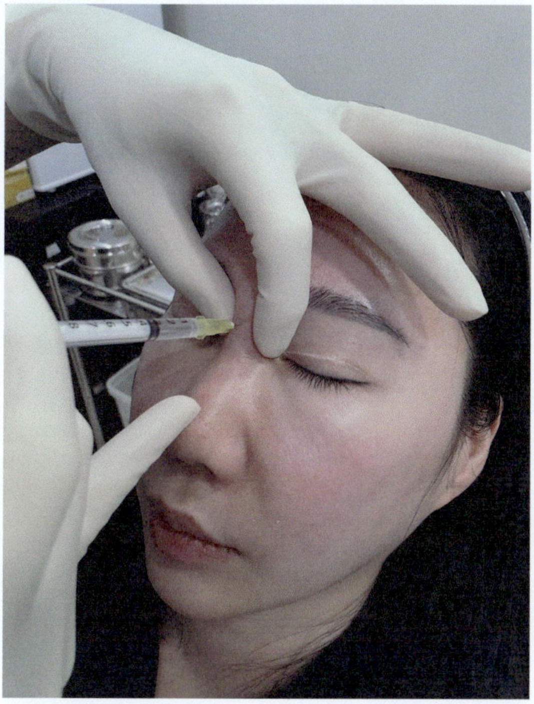

Fig. 3.18 Hyaluronidase injection at widening nose induced by previously HA injection

4 h after injection. But author recommends to inject HA filler again 1–2 days after injecting hyaluronidase after careful observation of hyaluronidase effect (Fig. 3.18).

3.5.4 Pre- and Postoperative Photograph

It is recommended to inject hard filler such as Lorient No. 6 at dorsum area and it is recommended to inject small amount of smooth filler such as No. 2 at nasal tip (Figs. 3.19, 3.20, 3.21, and 3.22).

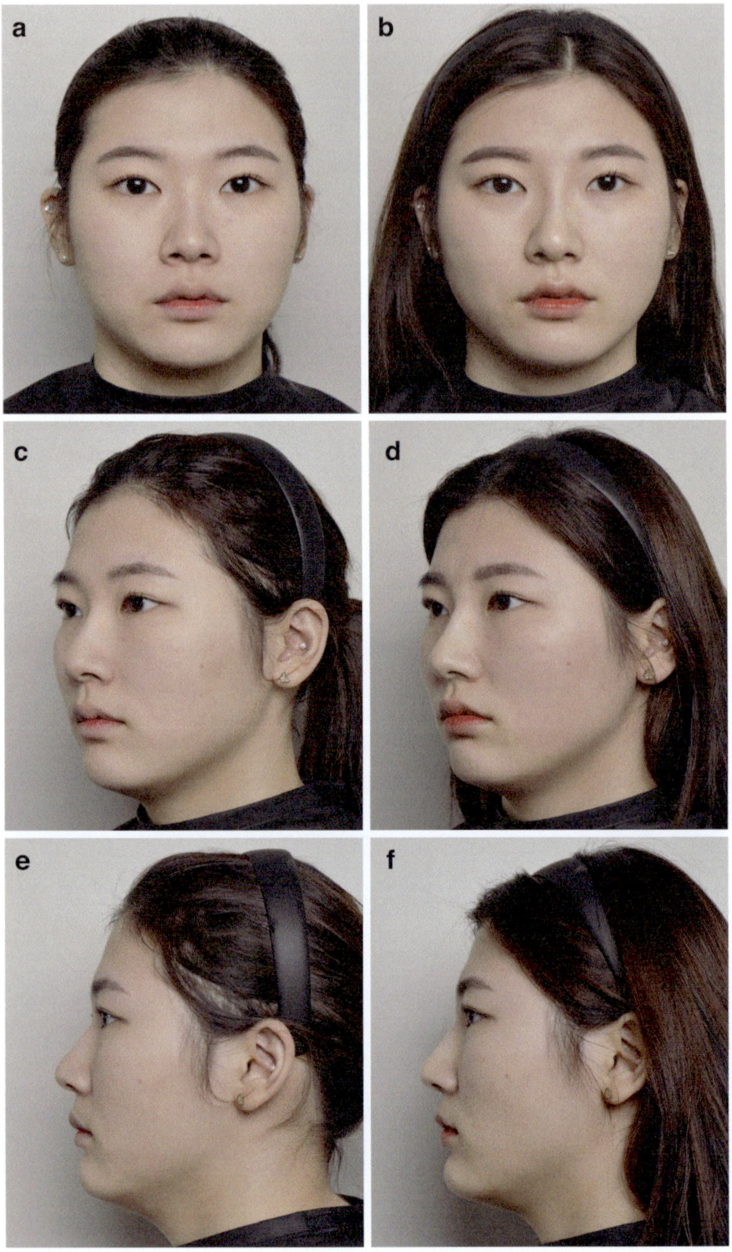

Fig. 3.19 Pre- and postoperative view of nose augmentation. Lorient No. 6 0.5 cc at supraperiosteal layer and No. 2 0.2 cc at nasal tip. (**a**) Preoperative frontal view. (**b**) Postoperative 2 days frontal view. (**c**) Preoperative three-quarter view. (**d**) Postoperative 2 days three-quarter view. (**e**) Preoperative lateral view. (**f**) Postoperative 2 days lateral view

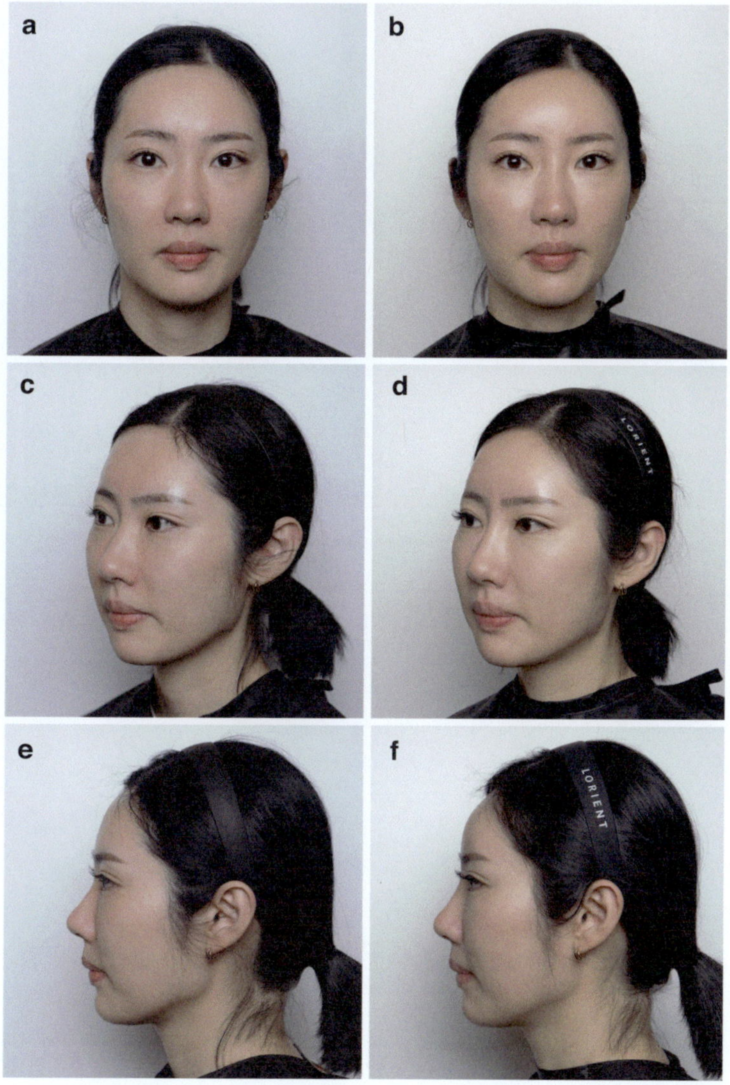

Fig. 3.20 Pre- and postoperative view of a 36-year-old female with nose augmentation. Lorient No. 6 0.6 cc at supraperiosteal layer for mild hump. (**a**) Preoperative frontal view. (**b**) Postoperative 2 weeks frontal view. (**c**) Preoperative three-quarter view. (**d**) Postoperative 2 weeks three-quarter view. (**e**) Preoperative lateral view. (**f**) Postoperative 2 weeks lateral view

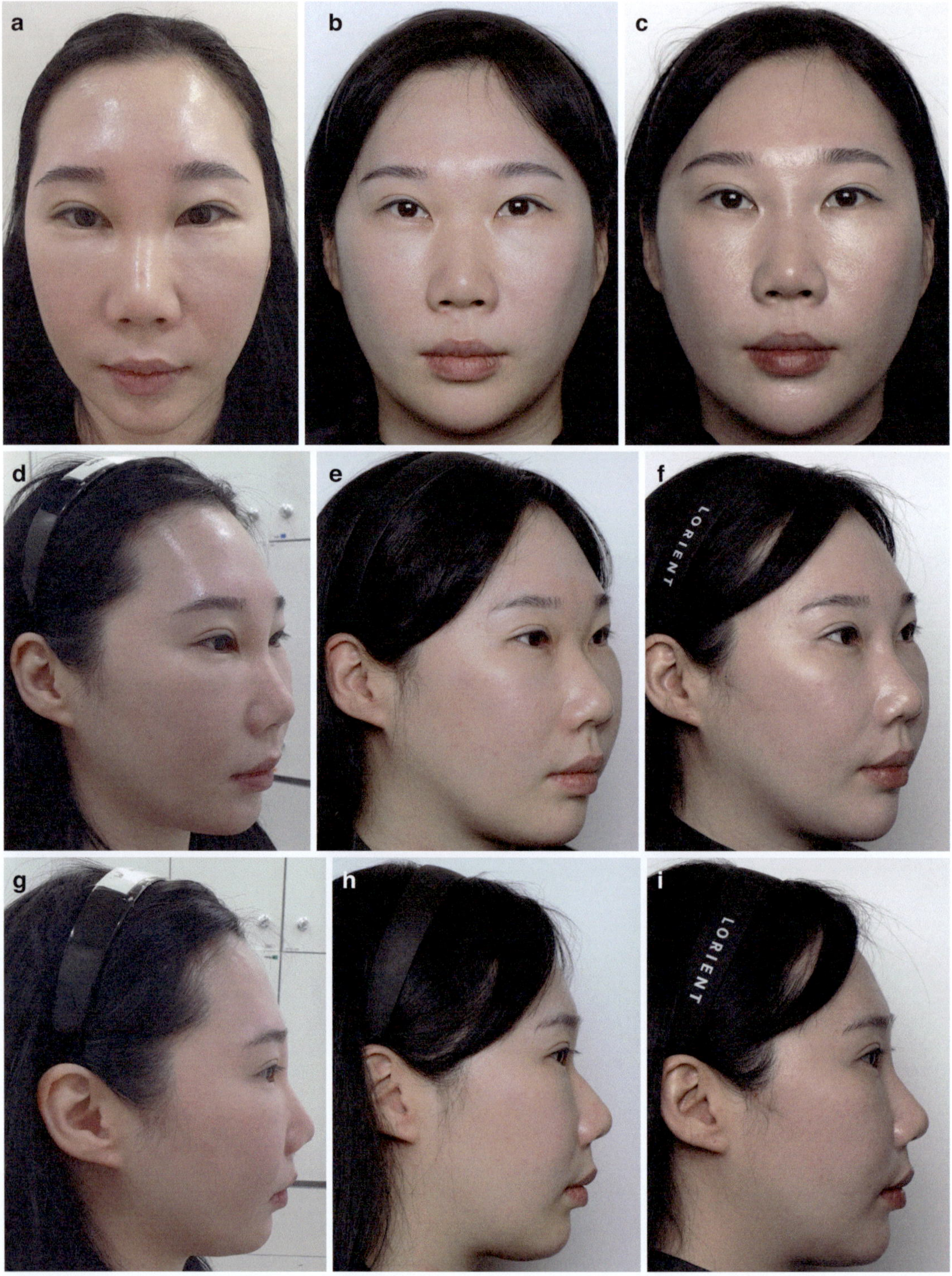

Fig. 3.21 Pre- and postoperative view of a 36-year-old female with widened nose correction. 0.5 cc of hyaluronidase injected and injected Lorient No. 6 0.8 cc at supraperiosteal layer 2 days after. (**a**) Preoperative frontal view. (**b**) Post hyaluronidase injection 2 days frontal view and preoperative HA filler injection. (**c**) Post HA filler injection 2 weeks frontal view. (**d**) Preoperative three-quarter view. (**e**) Post hyaluronidase injection 2 days three-quarter view and preoperative HA filler injection. (**f**) Post HA filler injection 2 weeks three-quarter view. (**g**) Preoperative lateral view. (**h**) Post hyaluronidase injection 2 days lateral view and preoperative HA filler injection. (**i**) Post HA filler injection 2 weeks lateral view

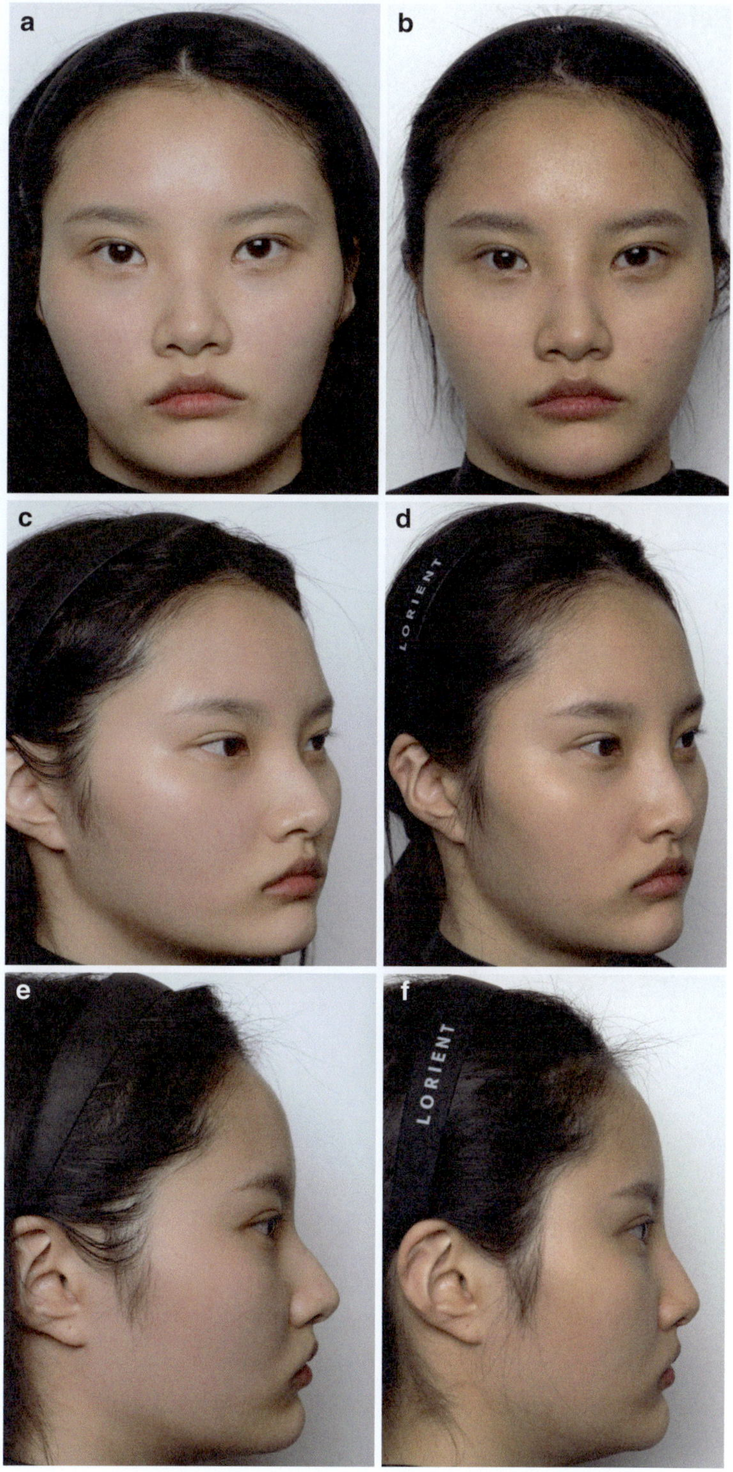

Fig. 3.22 Pre- and postoperative view of a 25-year-old female with nose augmentation. Lorient No. 6 0.5 cc at supraperiosteal layer for mild hump. (**a**) Preoperative frontal view. (**b**) Postoperative 2 weeks frontal view. (**c**) Preoperative three-quarter view. (**d**) Postoperative 2 weeks three-quarter view. (**e**) Preoperative lateral view. (**f**) Postoperative 2 weeks lateral view

References

1. Beleznay K, Carruthers JDA, Humphrey S, et al. Avoiding and treating blindness from fillers. Dermatologic Surg. 2015;41(10):1097–117.
2. Beleznay K, Carruthers JDA, Humphrey S, et al. Update on avoiding and treating blindness from fillers: a recent review of the world literature. Aesthet Surg J. 2019;39(6):662–74.
3. Lee W. Hyaluronic acid filler injection guided by Doppler ultrasound. Arch Plast Surg. 2023;50(4):348–53. https://doi.org/10.1055/s-0043-1770078.
4. Lee W, Moon HJ, Kim JS, Yang EJ. Safe glabellar wrinkle correction with soft tissue filler using Doppler ultrasound. Aesthet Surg J. 2021;41(9):1081–9. https://doi.org/10.1093/asj/sjaa197.
5. Lee W. Five factors to consider before treatment of a hyaluronic acid filler-induced vascular complications. Arch Plast Surg. 2022;49(4):479–81. https://doi.org/10.1055/s-0042-1751102.
6. Lee W, Koh IS, Oh W, et al. Ocular complications of soft tissue filler injections: a review of literature. J Cosmet Dermatol. 2020;19(4):772–81.
7. Cong LY, Phothong W, Lee SH, et al. Topographic analysis of the supratrochlear artery and the supraorbital artery: implication for improving the safety of forehead augmentation. Plast Reconstr Surg. 2017;139(3):620e–7.
8. Lee W, Kim JS, Oh W, Koh IS, Yang EJ. Nasal dorsum augmentation using soft tissue filler injection. J Cosmet Dermatol. 2019;18(5):1254–60. https://doi.org/10.1111/jocd.13018.
9. Danks JJ, Dalgliesh JD, Ayton T. Cosmetic filler blindness: recovery after repeated hyaluronidase injections. Aesthet Surg J. 2022;42(4):411–6. https://doi.org/10.1093/asj/sjab334.

4 Ultrasound Guided Hyaluronic Acid Filler Injection: External Carotid Artery Territories

Contents

4.1 Introduction

It is relatively difficult for the external carotid artery branch territories filler injection to cause ocular blindness. However, few cases have been reported to date. Reports mention injections at the nasolabial fold area where the facial artery is located, as well as at the temple area, where the superficial temporal artery is located. These arteries are known as large-diameter arteries in the face and are anastomosed to the ophthalmic artery branches. Thus, even if it is the external carotid artery branches, it is recommended to detect the structure by Doppler ultrasound before performing hyaluronic acid filler injection. Furthermore, the facial and superficial temporal arteries are easily detected by Doppler ultrasonography. In this chapter, we will discuss findings following Doppler ultrasonography and the corresponding guided injection techniques.

4.2 Temple Augmentation

The temple area is one of the most complicated areas for filler injections because of its many layers; however, it is also one of the easiest areas to detect by ultrasound. The temple is defined as the distance from the superior temporal septum to the zygomatic arch. The layers are the skin, subcutaneous layer, superficial temporal fascia (STF), deep temporal fascia (DTF), temporalis muscle, and bone (Fig. 4.1). The DTF can be divided into superficial and deep layers with loose areolar tissue located between the two layers. Loose areolar tissue is divided into the innominate fascia, and the parotid temporal fascia depends on location [1].

The HA filler can be injected into the three locations of these multiple layers. Subcutaneous layer, space between the STF and DTF, and deep into the temporalis muscle layer. There are some

W. Lee, *Advances in Hyaluronic Acid Filler Injections*,
https://doi.org/10.1007/978-981-97-6528-7_4

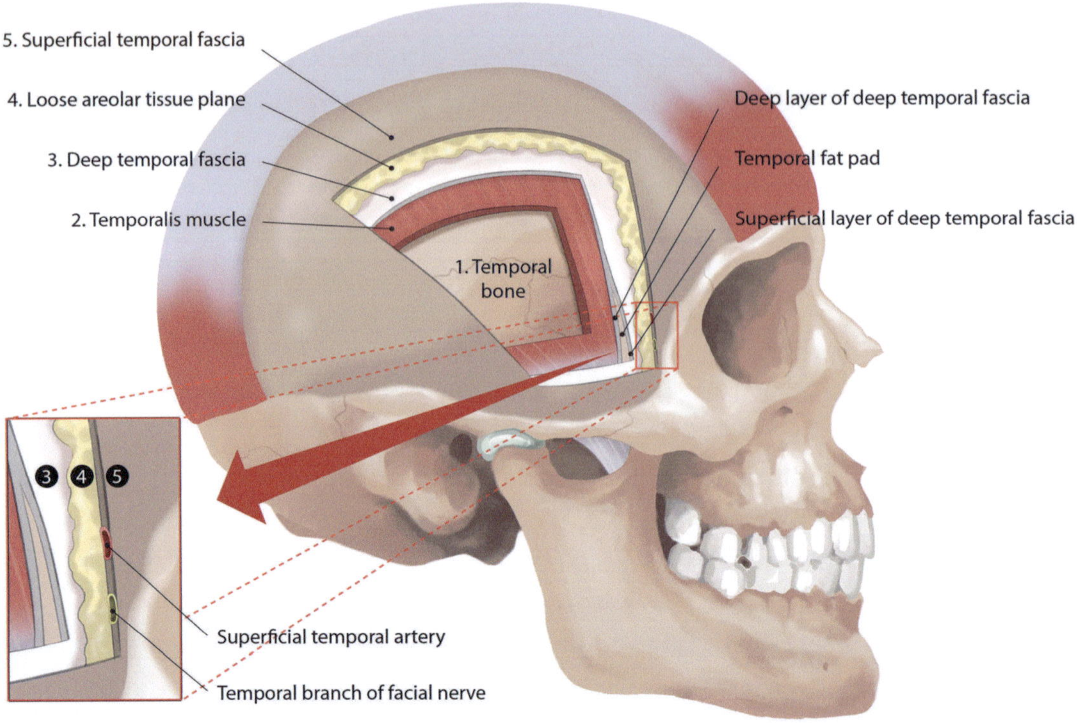

Fig. 4.1 Multiple layers of temple area

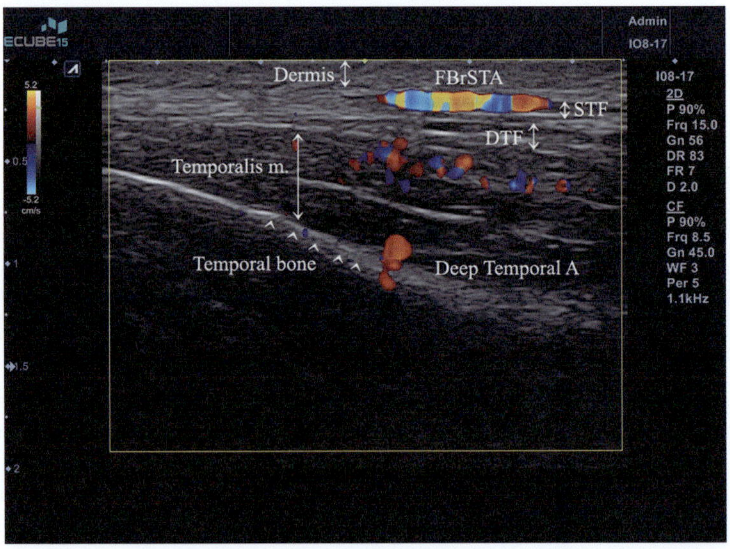

Fig. 4.2 Arteries at temple area. Frontal branch of superficial temporal artery (FBrSTA) and deep temporal artery anterior branch

considerations regarding deep-layer injection; therefore, the author usually injects in the space between the STF and DTF [2]. Deep-layer injections can cause damage of the deep temporal artery (Fig. 4.2).

Thus, when performing temple augmentation with HA filler, it is recommended to check the layers and arteries before injection to ensure safe delivery (Fig. 4.3).

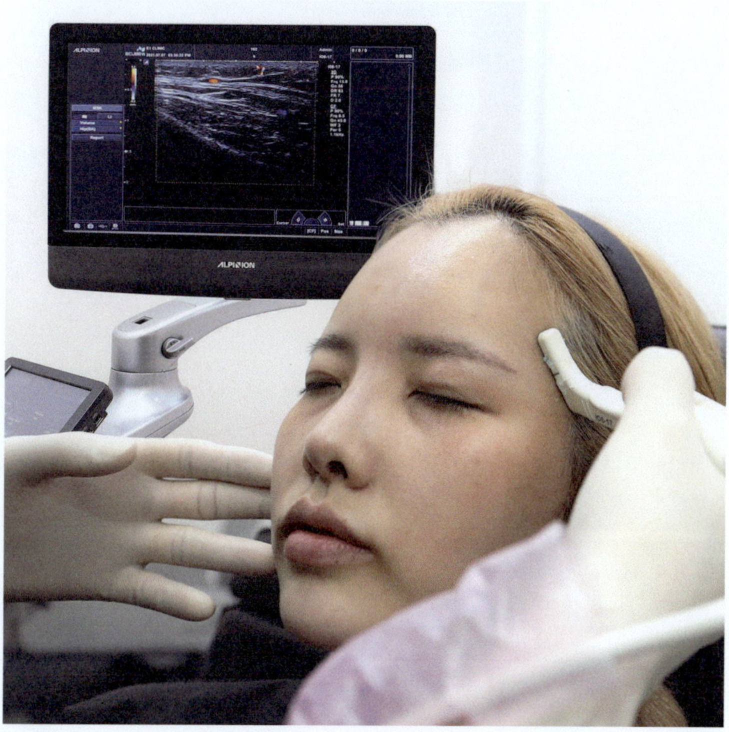

Fig. 4.3 Doppler ultrasound detection of the temple area

Table 4.1 Rheology of Lorient HA filler

Product	G′ (Pa)	G″ (Pa)	Complex viscosity (μ)	Tan delta	Cohesiveness (N)
Lorient No. 2	203	41	1,673,007	0.20	0.4401
Lorient No. 4	338	95	2,795,776	0.28	0.4237
Lorient No. 6	413	121	3,423,232	0.29	0.4454

Author uses No. 4 for temple augmentation

As described previously, the author uses the layer between the STF and DTF; thus, a hard filler is not needed. The author usually uses Lorient No. 4, which is the same HA filler used for forehead augmentation (Table 4.1).

First, Doppler ultrasound is performed to detect the arteries of the temple area and then create an entry point near the hairline. 21G cannula was used for gentle injections (Fig. 4.4a). Minimal resistance can occur during STF perforation using a cannula, and it can easily perforate. However, DTF have a harder structure and relatively hard resistance, making it difficult to perforate the DTF [3]. Thus, the cannula tip could easily be located between the STF and DTF, to inject the HA filler. At the end of the operation, it is recommended that the patient be in an upright position and the HA filler be injected by observing the final facial contour (Fig. 4.4b). When performing deep-layer injection, it is possible to inject more than 3 mL of HA filler on one side, but when injected in the space between the STF and DTF, generally less than 1.5 mL of HA filler is required (Figs. 4.5, 4.6, and 4.7).

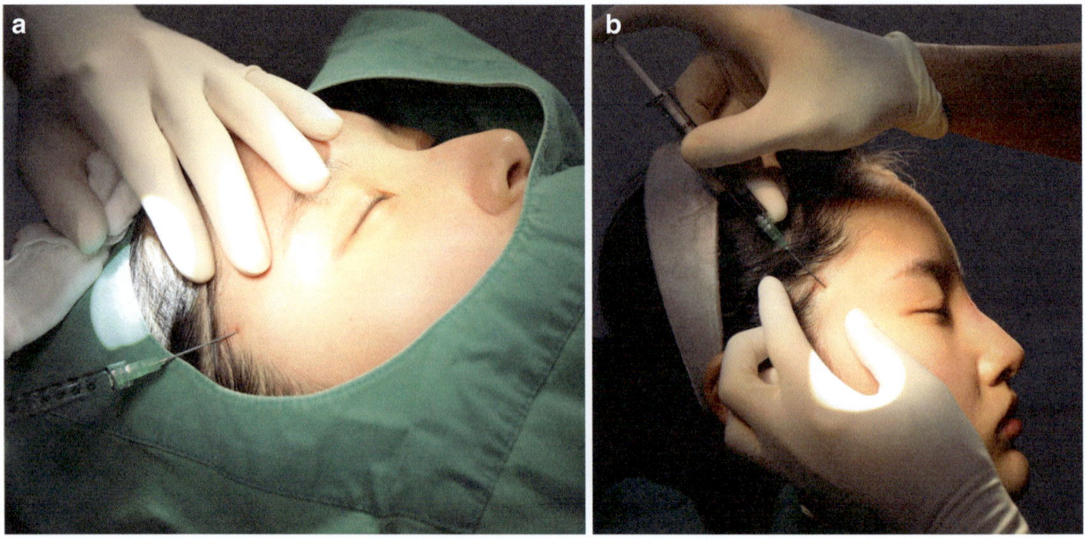

Fig. 4.4 HA fille injection at the temple area. (**a**) HA filler injected at the space between STF and DTF at supine position. (**b**) Patient in an upright position and additional injection for smooth facial contour

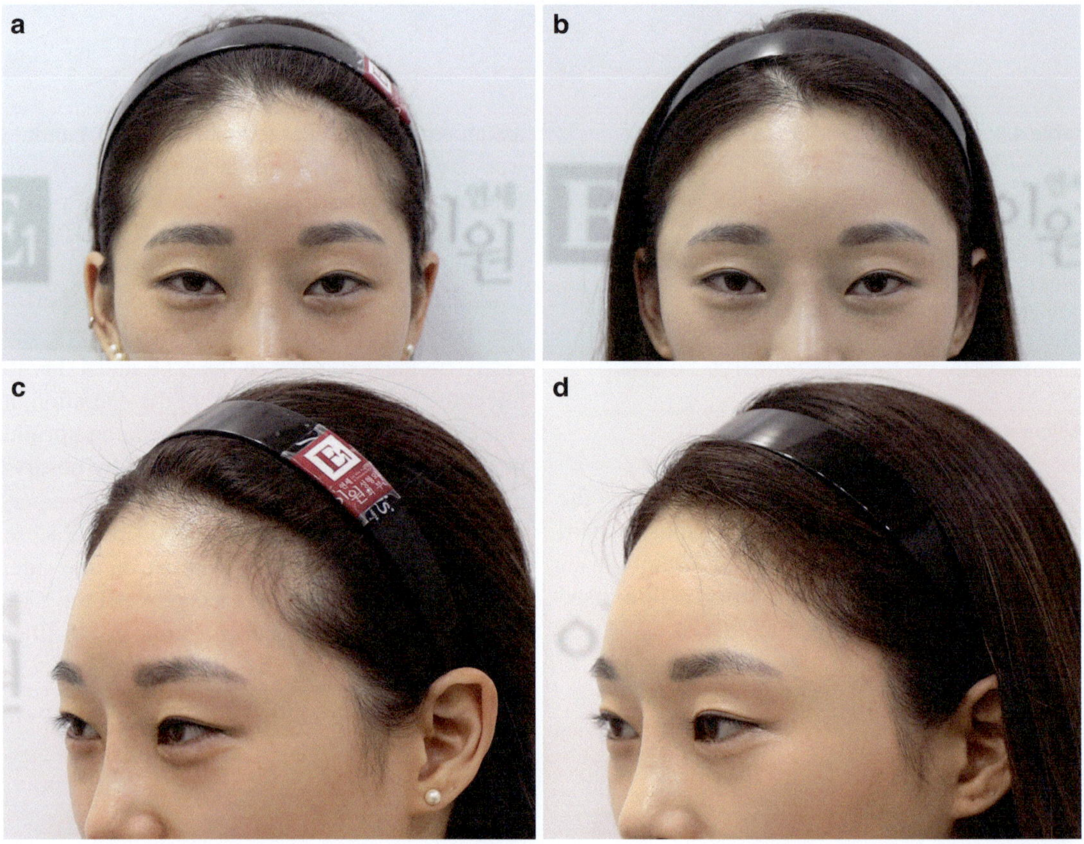

Fig. 4.5 A 29-year-old woman who underwent the injection of 1 cc of HA filler on one side of the temple. (**a**) Preoperative frontal view. (**b**) Postoperative 2 weeks frontal view. (**c**) Preoperative three-quarter view. (**d**) Postoperative 2 weeks three-quarter view

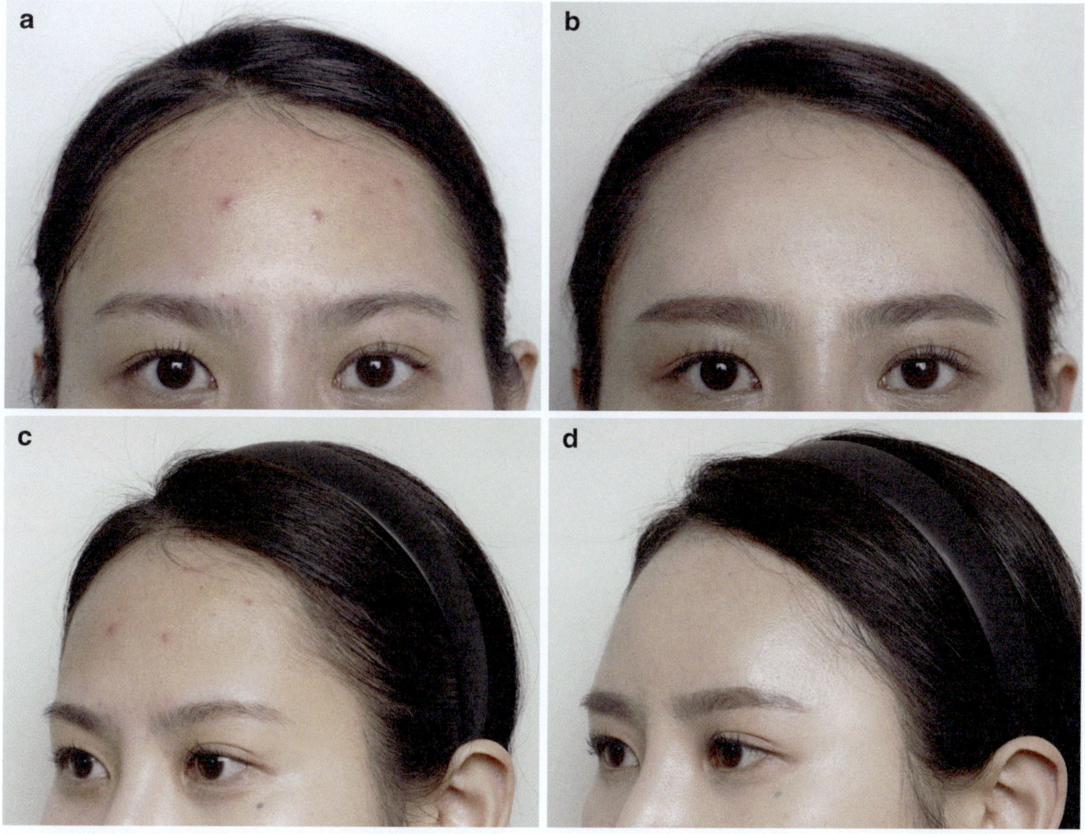

Fig. 4.6 A-23–year-old woman injected with 1 cc of HA filler on one side of temple. (**a**) Preoperative frontal view. (**b**) Postoperative 2 weeks frontal view. (**c**) Preoperative three-quarter view. (**d**) Postoperative 2 weeks three-quarter view

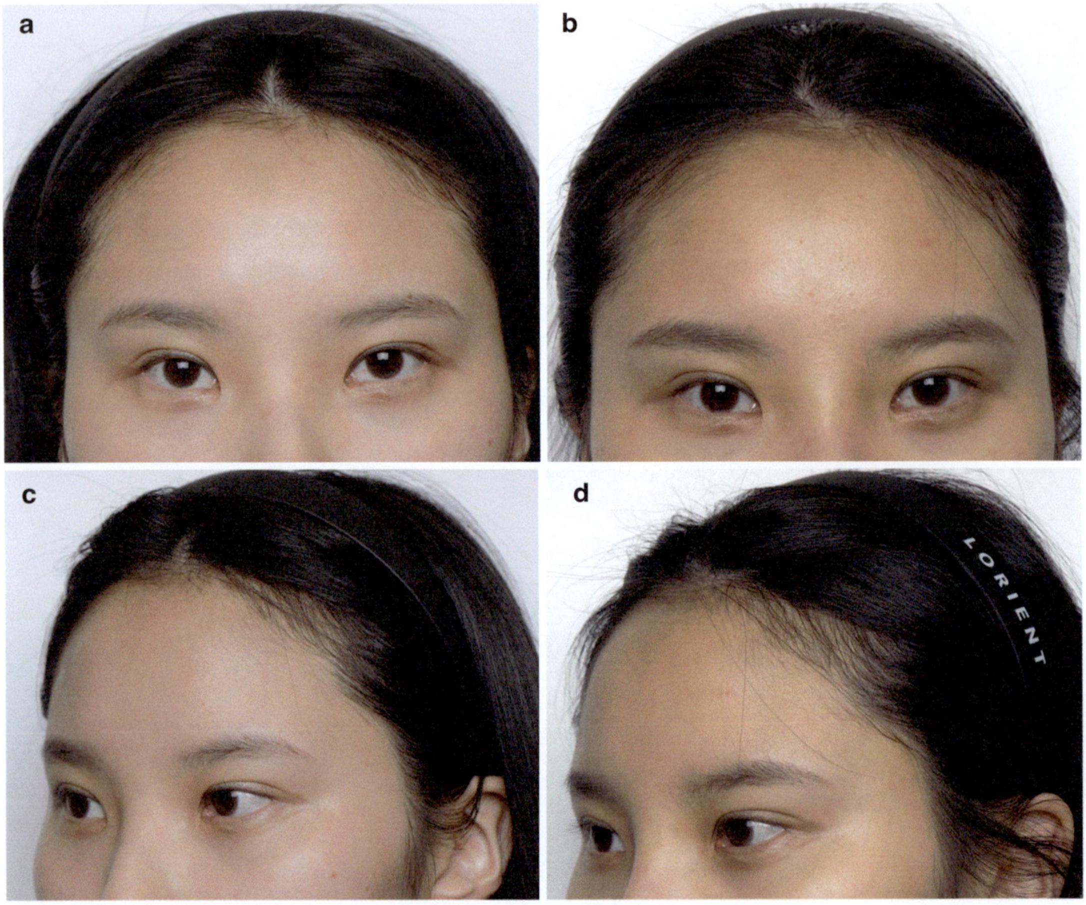

Fig. 4.7 A-25-year-old women injected with 1 cc of HA filler on one side of the temple. (**a**). Preoperative frontal view. (**b**) Postoperative 2 weeks frontal view. (**c**) Preoperative three-quarter view. (**d**) Postoperative 2 weeks three-quarter view

4.3 Nasolabial Fold Correction

Nasolabial fold correction is one of the most commonly performed HA filler injections. One of the most commonly used scale is the wrinkle severity rate scale (WSRS), which is based on nasolabial fold evaluation. Multiple etiologies of the nasolabial fold have been proposed, including the nasolabial fat, which is the superficial fat compartment that causes sagging of the face upon aging by decreasing dermal elasticity [4]. In addition, its etiology is decreasing deep medial cheek fat (DMCF) [5]. Ristow's space is a potential surgical space located between the DMCF and periosteum, and the injection of HA filler in this space is essential to correct the nasolabial fold. Repetitive lip elevator muscles can also perform nasolabial folding [6] (Fig. 4.8).

Successful nasolabial fold correction is achieved by deep and superficial layer injections. The relatively large diameter facial artery runs along the nasolabial fold area; therefore, detecting the arteries using Doppler ultrasound before injection is recommended (Fig. 4.9).

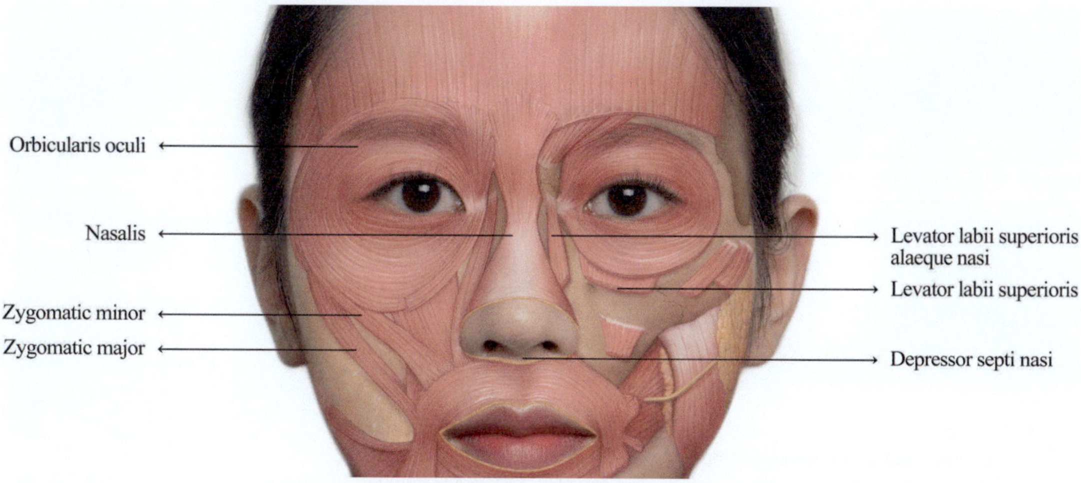

Fig. 4.8 Facial muscle consideration for nasolabial fold injection

Fig. 4.9 Doppler ultrasound image of the nasolabial fold area

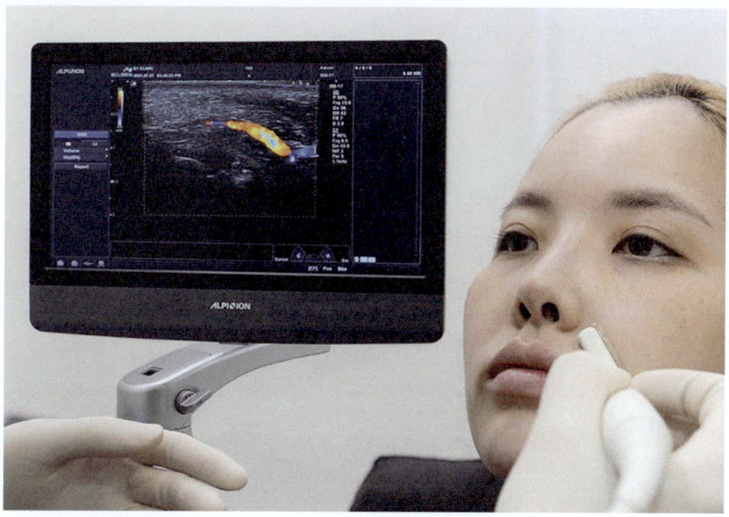

A nasolabial fold correction can be performed by needle or cannula injections. Perpendicular injection using a needle is a commonly performed procedure; the needle tip should be located in the supraperiosteal layer. Despite being a controversial technique, the aspiration test is recommended rather than not using, especially in the nasolabial fold area. Using cannula is not a completely safer technique either; yet, Doppler ultrasonography is to be conducted before injecting the HA filler, either by a needle or cannula. The cannula tip should also be located in the supraperiosteal layer, and be gently injected into the DMCF (Fig. 4.10). After deep injection, it is recommended to inject a minimal amount of HA filler into the subdermal layer to correct the wrinkles (Fig. 4.11). The nasolabial fold cannot disappear; therefore, improving the fold should be the goal of nasolabial HA filler injection (Figs. 4.12 and 4.13). When the HA filler is injected into the upper portion of the nasolabial fold, lateral nasal artery occlusion develops.

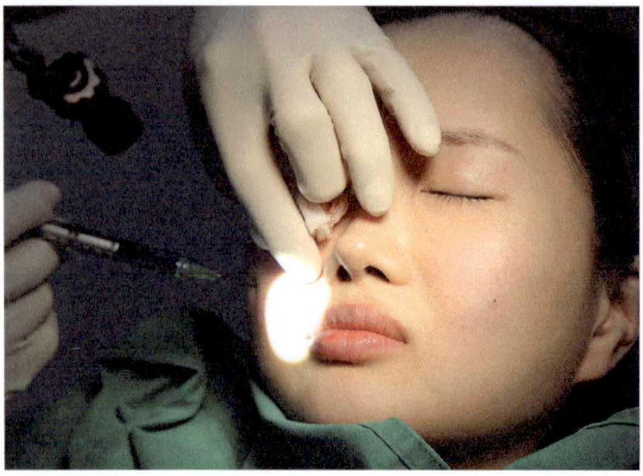

Fig. 4.10 Lateral approach to nasolabial fold by cannula performed. The cannula tip should be located in the supraperiosteal layer followed by gentle injection of Lorient No. 4 or No. 6

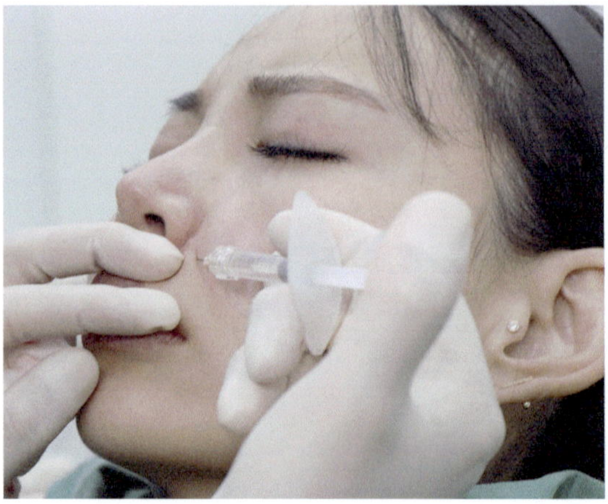

Fig. 4.11 Subdermal injection of Lorient No. 2 HA filler for correcting nasolabial fold wrinkle

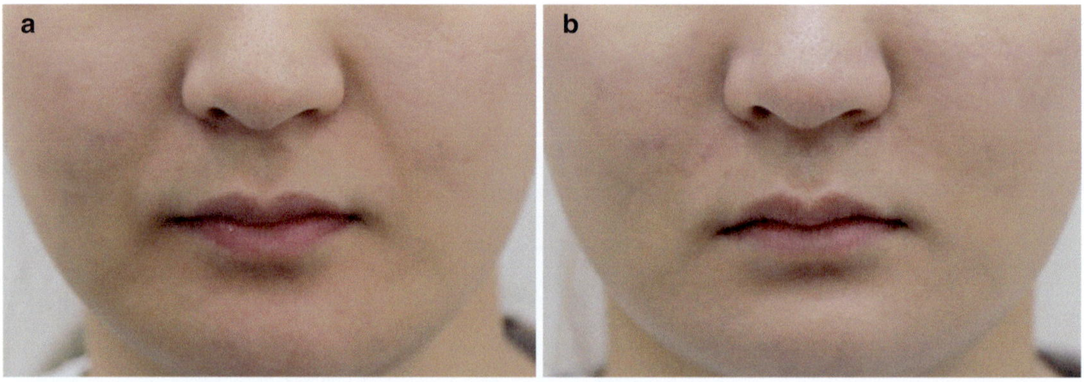

Fig. 4.12 A-27-year-old woman underwent 1 cc implantation at one side of the nasolabial fold. (**a**) Preoperative. (**b**) Postoperative 2 weeks

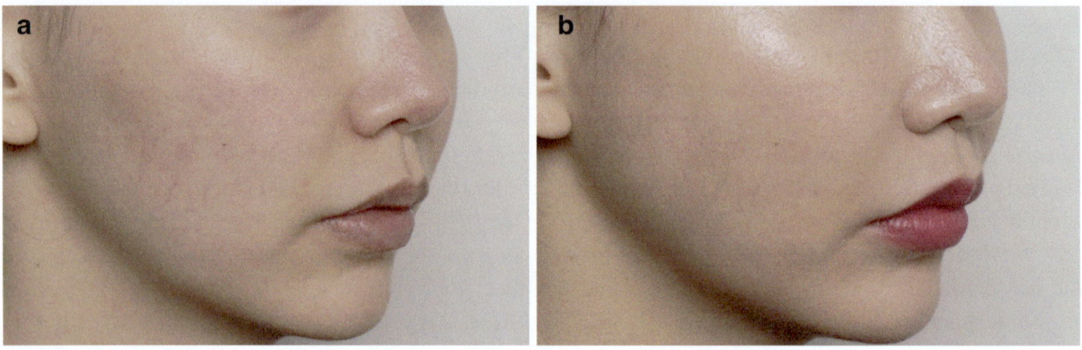

Fig. 4.13 A-35-year-old women undergoing 0.5 cc implantation at one side of the nasolabial fold. (**a**) Preoperative. (**b**) Postoperative 2 weeks

4.4 Lip Augmentation

The lip contour becomes more ambiguous upon aging; thus, HA filler lip injection can make the lip more prominent and younger in appearance. The ideal proportion of the upper and lower lips is 1:1.5, and it is recommended to perform lip injection in the upright position. Doppler ultrasound detection of the superior and inferior labial arteries before HA filler injection is a safer method. However, these arteries tend to run near the mucosa, and lip injection is usually performed on the superficial layer; thus, the lips are a relatively safer area (Fig. 4.14). Usually, lip injections by a needle are safe (Fig. 4.15). Preoperative and postoperative photographs are shown (Figs. 4.16, 4.17, and 4.18).

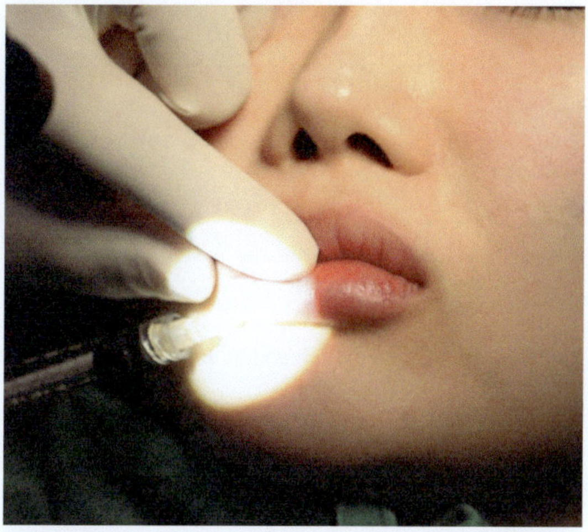

Fig. 4.15 Lower lip augmentation. Relatively large amount of HA filler is injected compared to the upper lip

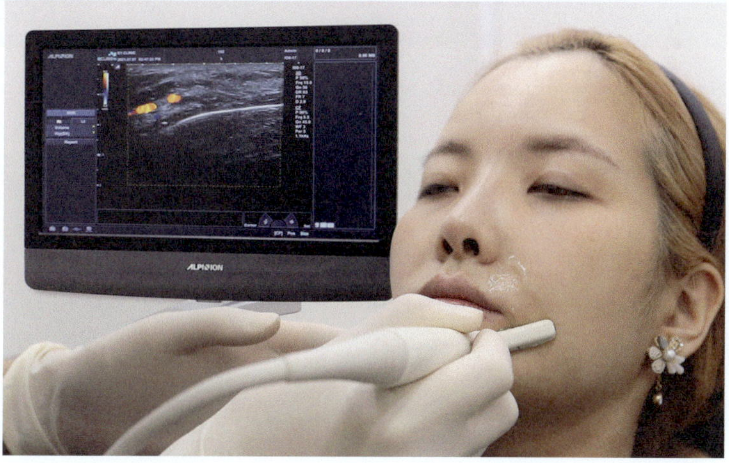

Fig. 4.14 Inferior labial artery Doppler ultrasound finding

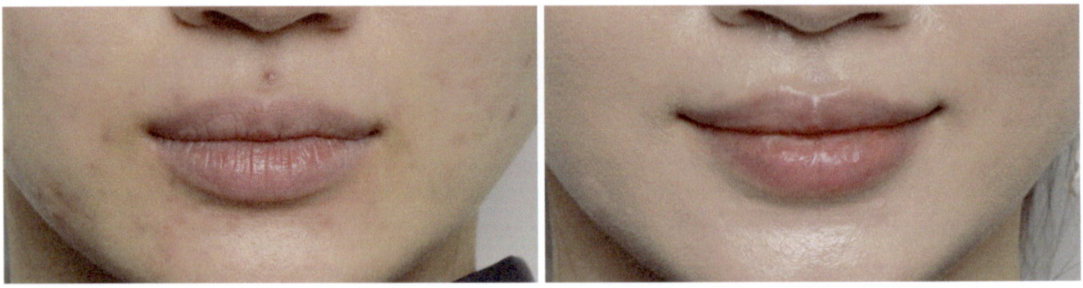

Fig. 4.16 Lip augmentation and mouth corner lifting. Preoperative and postoperative 2 weeks

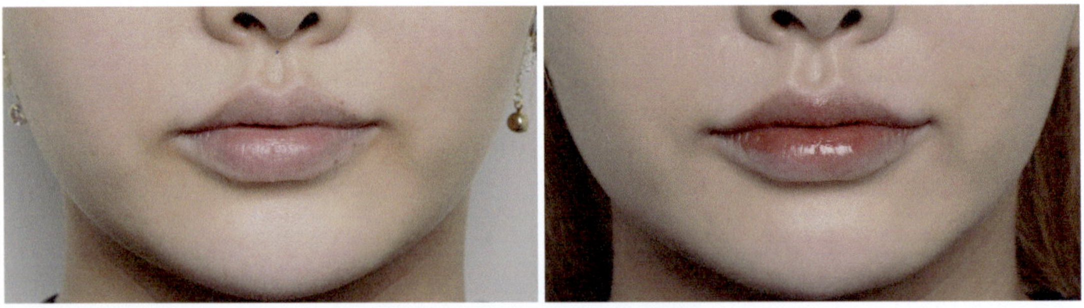

Fig. 4.17 Lip augmentation and mouth corner lifting. Preoperative and postoperative 2 weeks

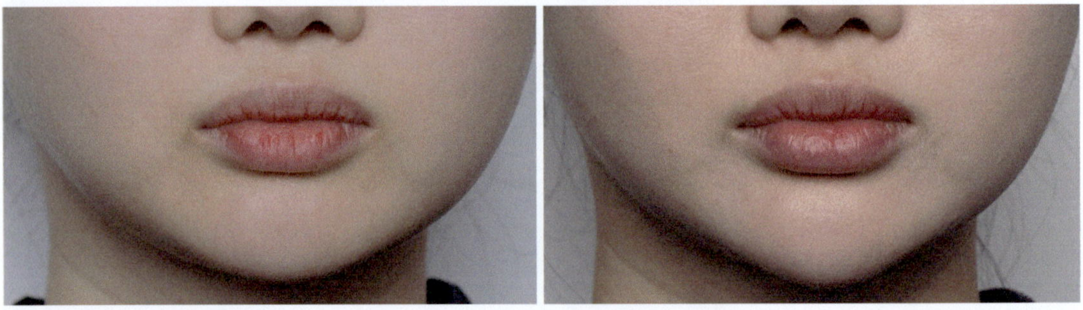

Fig. 4.18 Lip augmentation. Preoperative and postoperative 2 weeks

4.5 Chin Augmentation

Mouth protrusions do not have a good aesthetic appearance. It usually depends on the Rickettes' line, which is a virtual line extending from the end of the chin to the nose tip [7]. Traditionally, bone surgeries such as genioplasty or silicone implant insertion have been performed for chin elongation. However, injecting HA filler in the chin area is a very simple method compared to the traditional operation, and minimal change can be more attractive.

The chin area is relatively safe; however, its relationship with the mentalis muscle should be considered. The mentalis muscle retains the lower lip and shows a cobblestone appearance when contracted; therefore, botulinum toxin injection is required before HA filler injection. The author recommends injecting multiple layers rather than a bolus injection (Figs. 4.19 and 4.20).

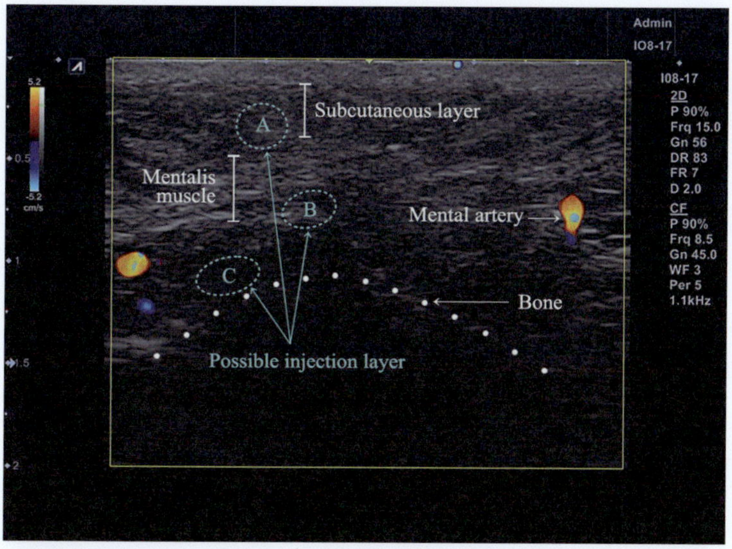

Fig. 4.19 Ultrasound finding of the chin area and possible layer of chin augmentation. (A) Superficial fat (mental fat compartment). (B) Submentalis layer (submentalis fat). (C) Supraperiosteal layer (submentalis fat)

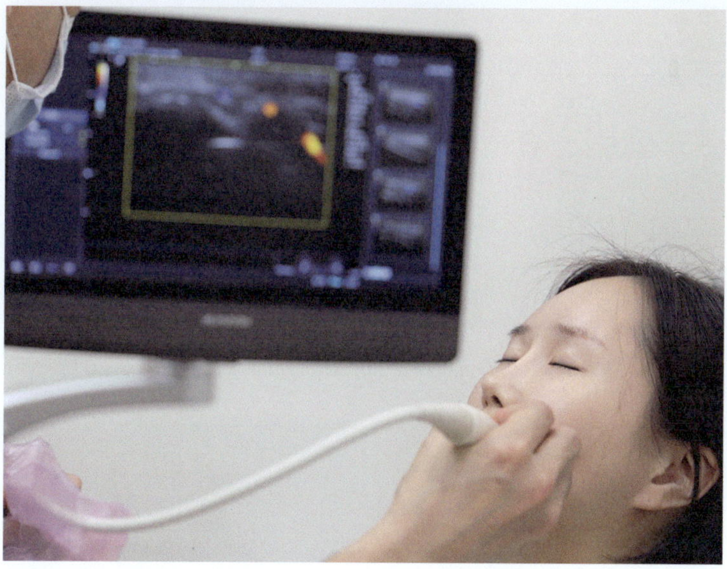

Fig. 4.20 Doppler ultrasonography of the chin area

The most high G′ HA filler is recommended (Table 4.2).

Midline injection into the chin area is a useful technique for enhancing the chin. The submental artery branch may run midline, so that the entry point can be made laterally using a cannula. The most important factor in chin injection is deciding whether to elongate or protrude the chin. In addition, maintaining symmetry is crucial (Figs. 4.21, 4.22, and 4.23).

Table 4.2 Rheology of HA filler

Product	G′ (Pa)	G″ (Pa)	Complex viscosity (μ)	Tan delta	Cohesiveness (N)
Lorient No. 2	203	41	1,673,007	0.20	0.4401
Lorient No. 4	338	95	2,795,776	0.28	0.4237
Lorient No. 6	413	121	3,423,232	0.29	0.4454

For the chin, No. 6 is recommended

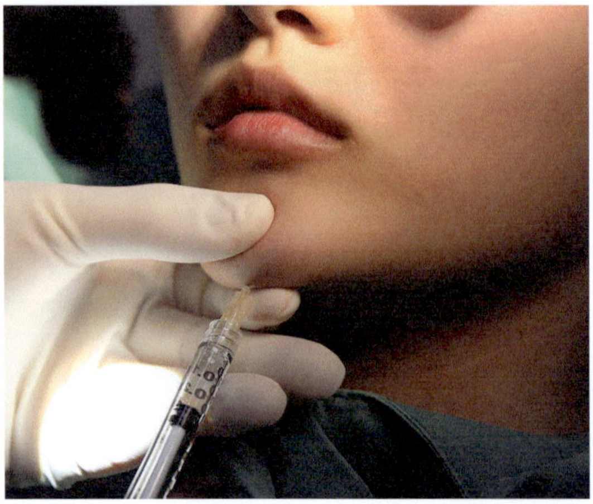

Fig. 4.21 Chin augmentation by HA filler

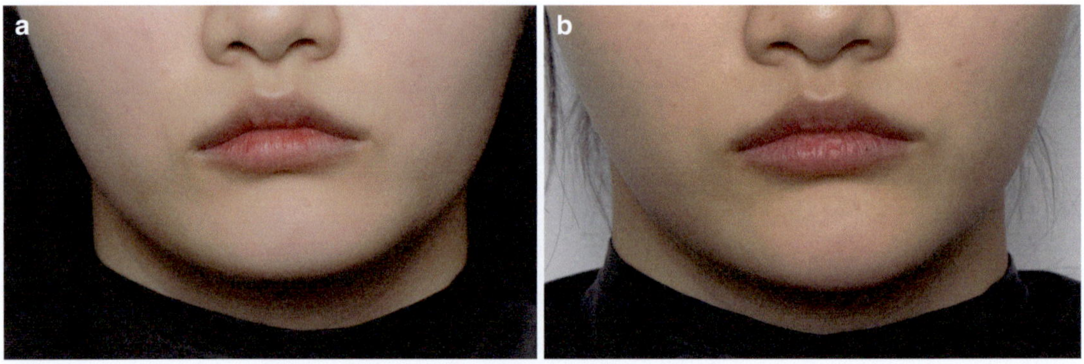

Fig. 4.22 A 25-year-old female was injected Lorient No. 6 0.5 cc. (**a**) Preoperative. (**b**) Postoperative 2 weeks

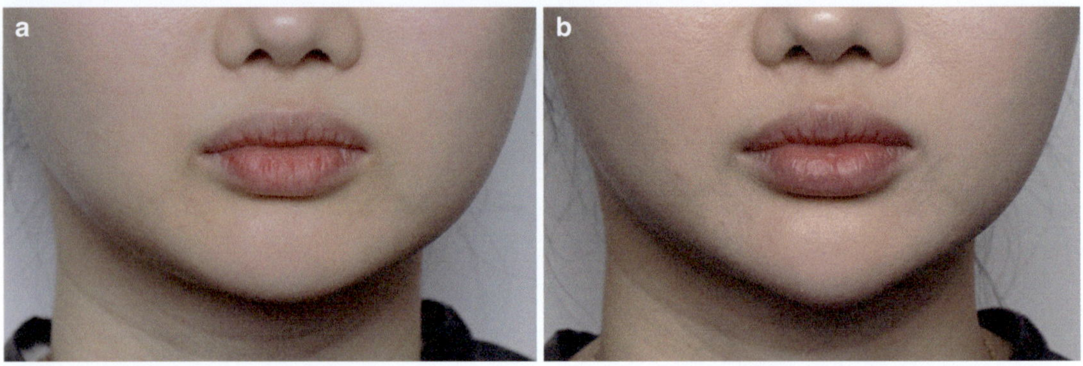

Fig. 4.23 A 37-year-old female injected with Lorient No. 6 0.9 cc. (**a**) Preoperative. (**b**) Postoperative 2 weeks

4.6 Midface Augmentation

The midface constitutes complex structures, including the skin, tear trough, orbicularis retaining ligament, zygomaticocutaneous ligament, suborbicularis oculi fat (SOOF) and the orbicularis oculi muscle. Filler injections to the midface are usually done simultaneously at multiple locations at once. For example, the tear trough, anterior malar, and lateral cheek are corrected concomitantly. The total amount of the filler should be considered. The nasojugal groove appears in complex structures such as the tear trough ligament, orbital septal fat, and border between the preseptal and orbital portions of the orbicularis oculi muscle. The orbicularis retaining ligament can be divided into the medial and lateral sides by the midpupillary line, and the medial side develops to become tighter and of hard structure. The medial side is a tight structure because the orbicularis retaining ligament and the zygomaticocutaneous ligament tend to aggregate on the medial side [8].

When orbital fat is extruded, transconjunctival or transcutaneous surgical removal is required. However, if only the nasojugal groove is present, filler injection can yield good results. When muscle fibers extend tightly to the orbital rim or tear trough ligaments are tightly attached, good aesthetic results cannot be achieved only by HA filler injection. Surgical correction is the only available treatment option. Usually, muscle fibers are not attached to the orbital rim tightly and good aesthetic correction can be performed using an HA filler injection.

One of the common problems associated with periorbital HA filler injections is edema. It is known as post-hyaluronic acid recurrent eyelid edema (PHAREE) and is associated with the lymphatics [9]. It is important to understand the structure of the lower eyelid and to not overfill the HA filler.In addition, the pathway of the angular artery and Doppler ultrasound can be useful for detecting the artery (Figs. 4.24 and 4.25).

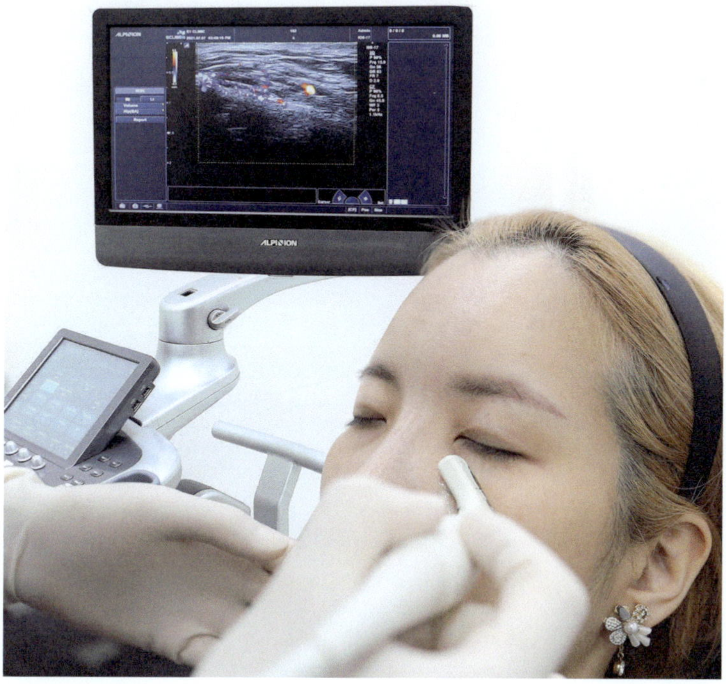

Fig. 4.24 Doppler ultrasound detection of the angular artery at the nasojugal groove area

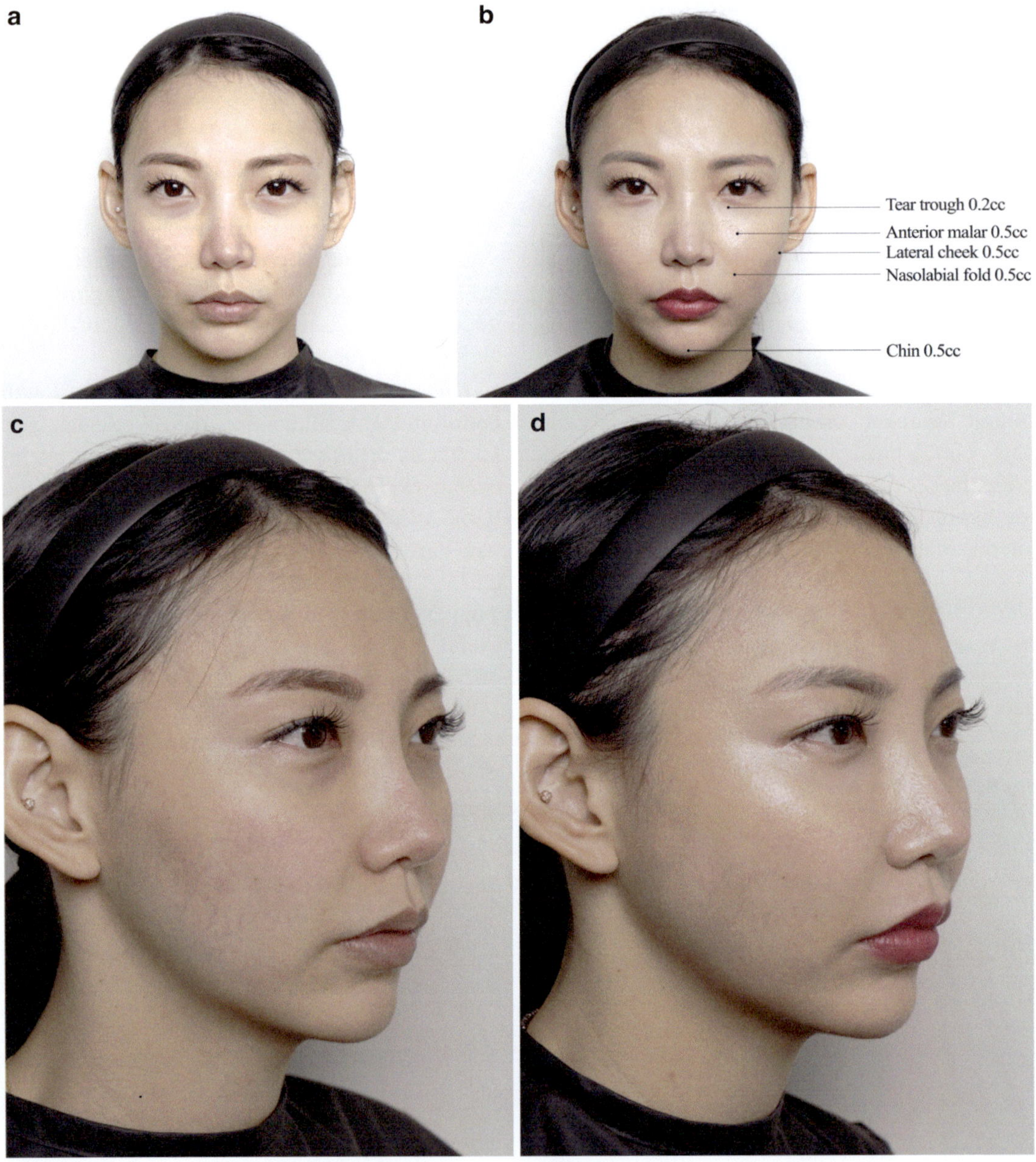

Fig. 4.25 A 35-year-old woman undergoing midface augmentation. (**a**) Preoperative frontal view. (**b**) Postoperative 2 weeks frontal view. (**c**) Preoperative three-quarter view. (**d**) Postoperative 2 weeks three-quarter view

References

1. Davidge KM, van Furth WR, Agur A, Cusimano M. Naming the soft tissue layers of the temporoparietal region: unifying anatomic terminology across surgical disciplines. Neurosurgery. 2010;67(3 Suppl Operative):ons120-9.
2. Lee W, Park JW, Yang EJ. Temple augmentation by injecting a hyaluronic acid filler between the superficial and deep temporal fasciae. J Cosmet Dermatol. 2022;21(10):4313–8. https://doi.org/10.1111/jocd.15004.
3. Lee KL, Hong GW, Lee W, Kim HJ. Comparative study of the penetration force between the superficial and deep temporal fascia for easier temple augmentation technique using hyaluronic acid filler. J Plast Reconstr Aesthet Surg. 2023;77:271–3. https://doi.org/10.1016/j.bjps.2022.12.005.
4. Ezure T, Amano S. Involvement of upper cheek sagging in nasolabial fold formation. Skin Res Technol. 2012;18(3):259–64. https://doi.org/10.1111/j.1600-0846.2011.00567.x.
5. Rohrich RJ, Pessa JE, Ristow B. The youthful cheek and the deep medial fat compartment. Plast Reconstr Surg. 2008;121(6):2107–12. https://doi.org/10.1097/PRS.0b013e31817123c6.
6. Beer GM, Manestar M, Mihic-Probst D. The causes of the nasolabial crease: a histomorphological study. Clin Anat. 2013;26(2):196–203. https://doi.org/10.1002/ca.22100.
7. Ricketts RM. Perspectives in the clinical application of cephalometrics. The first fifty years. Angle Orthod. 1981;51(2):115–50. https://doi.org/10.1043/0003-3219(1981)051<0115:PITCAO>2.0.CO;2.
8. Wong CH, Mendelson B. Facial soft-tissue spaces and retaining ligaments of the midcheek: defining the premaxillary space. Plast Reconstr Surg. 2013;132(1):49–56. https://doi.org/10.1097/PRS.0b013e3182910a57.
9. Karlin J, et al. Post-hyaluronic acid recurrent eyelid edema: pathophysiologic mechanisms and a proposed treatment protocol. Aesthet Surg J Open Forum. 2023;5:ojad102.

Hyaluronic Acid Filler Analysis: Nuclear Magnetic Resonance (NMR)

5

Contents

5.1 Introduction

In this chapter, we will discuss about the crosslinker in hyaluronic acid (HA) fillers, which is known for a possible cause of delayed inflammatory reactions. HA filler is composed of HA and a crosslinker, usually 1,4-butanediol diglycidyl ether (BDDE). However, not all the BDDE crosslinks between the two HA chains occur optimally. Improperly crosslinked BDDE can be detected by nuclear magnetic resonance (NMR), and the results are described in this chapter.

5.2 Hyaluronic Acid Filler Structure

HA fillers have the naturally occurring component of HA, which is a disaccharide composed of acetylglucosamine and glucuronic acid (Fig. 5.1). These HA do not different across species; therefore, mass manufacturing uses bacteria-based HA. Hyaluronidase also exists as a component of the human body to degrade HA normally [1].

Thus, the HA filler is composed of HA and a crosslinker. Various crosslinkers are used but

W. Lee, *Advances in Hyaluronic Acid Filler Injections*,
https://doi.org/10.1007/978-981-97-6528-7_5

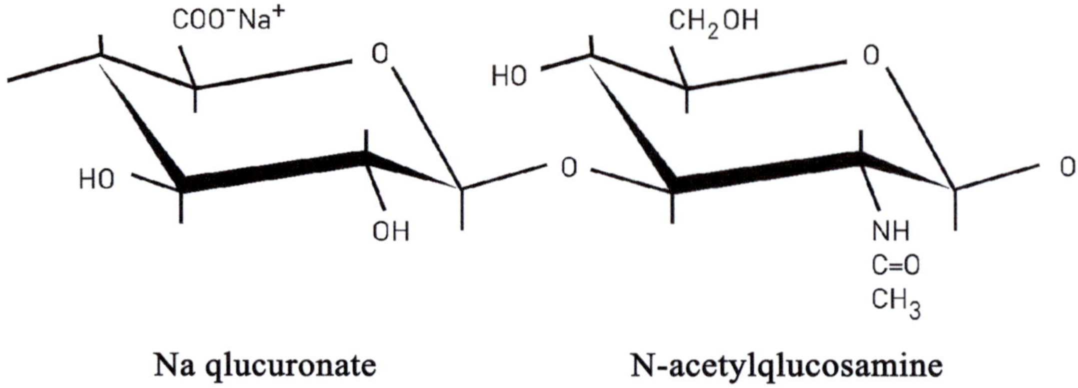

Fig. 5.1 Hyaluronic acid molecules (glucuronic acid and *N*-acetylglucosamine)

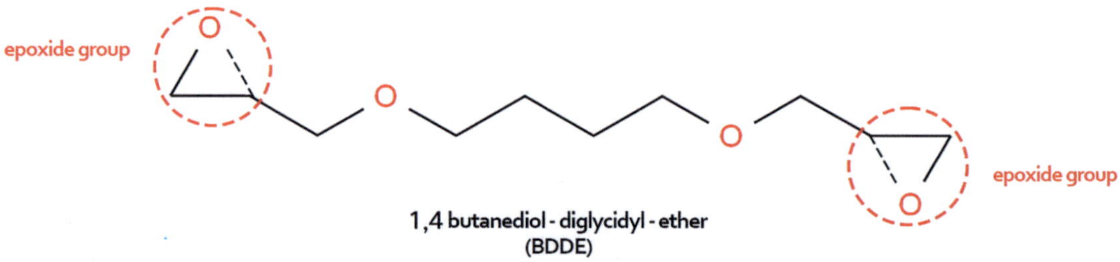

Fig. 5.2 Molecular structure of BDDE

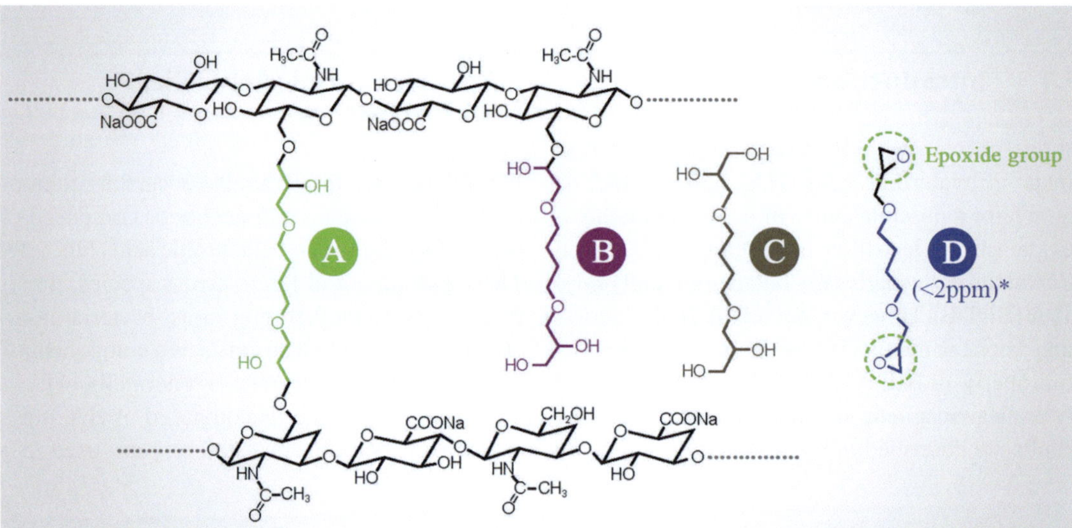

Fig. 5.3 Four different types of BDDE. (A) Proper crosslinked. (B) Pendant type. (C) BDPE. (D) Native

BDDE (Fig. 5.2) is commonly used. HA and BDDE are mixed and called the "reaction" process.

In this process, the BDDE epoxide ring should be opened such that the HA hydroxyl chain crosslinks with the ether bond. Yet sometimes optimal crosslinks fail, which form, what is known as the "pendant" type [2]. Following the mixing of HA with BDDE, BDDE exists as four different forms (Fig. 5.3).

When the BDDE epoxide rings are opened, BDDE changes as 1,4-butanediol di-(propan-2,3-diolyl) ether (BDPE) which is C in Fig. 5.3. Thus, BDDE is D of Fig. 5.3 and BDPE is denoted as C in Fig. 5.3. Types B and C did not properly act as crosslinks, and type A was the only type that acted as an appropriate crosslink.

Then, how can A, B, C, and D be determined? The D-type can be determined by gas chromatography. Generally, manufactured HA fillers should be detected less than 2 ppm. The question remains the amount of type B and/or type C.

5.3 Hyaluronic Acid Filler Impurities Detection: NMR Analysis

Various test methods have been proposed to detect the amounts of type A and B. Among various tests, NMR is one of the most reliable. NMR is used to detect specific molecules. Usually, carbon or hydrogen bonds are detected in organic chemical analyses. As described previously, HA is composed of N-acetylglucosamine and glucuronic acid. While BDDE is composed of carbon and hydrogen. Thus, NMR can detect the structure of the components of HA fillers. The HA filler can be degraded by chondroitinase and different molecules arise after degradation (Fig. 5.4).

As described previously, the HA filler is composed of HA and BDDE by four different types of residues, and when the HA filler is degraded by chondroitinase, multiple structures are seen (Fig. 5.5).

These structures are composed of carbon and hydrogen atoms. Therefore, NMR spectroscopy could be used to detect their specific structures. Structural analysis using hydrogen is referred to as ^{1}H NMR, and when carbon is used, it is called ^{13}C NMR. The atomic number should be odd because a spin proton can occur. Typically, NMR machines operate at 200–600 MHz, and the number indicates the hydrogen resonance frequency. When the frequency is high, the magnetic field is higher, and the spectrum resolution is better. The AscendTM 600 MHz spectrometer (Bruker Co.) is widely used to detect high-resolution results. Almost every organic component can be analyzed by a 200–600 MHz machine. For NMR with frequencies below 300 MHz, permanent magnets and electromagnets are used instead of expensive

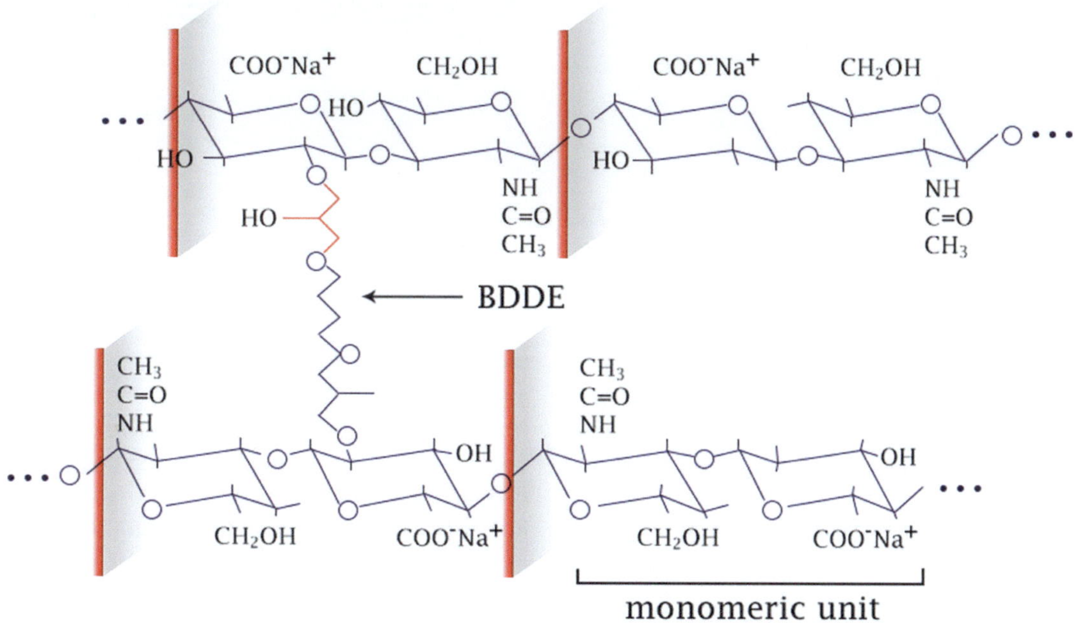

Fig. 5.4 Crosslinked hyaluronic acid filler can be degraded by chondroitinase (red line)

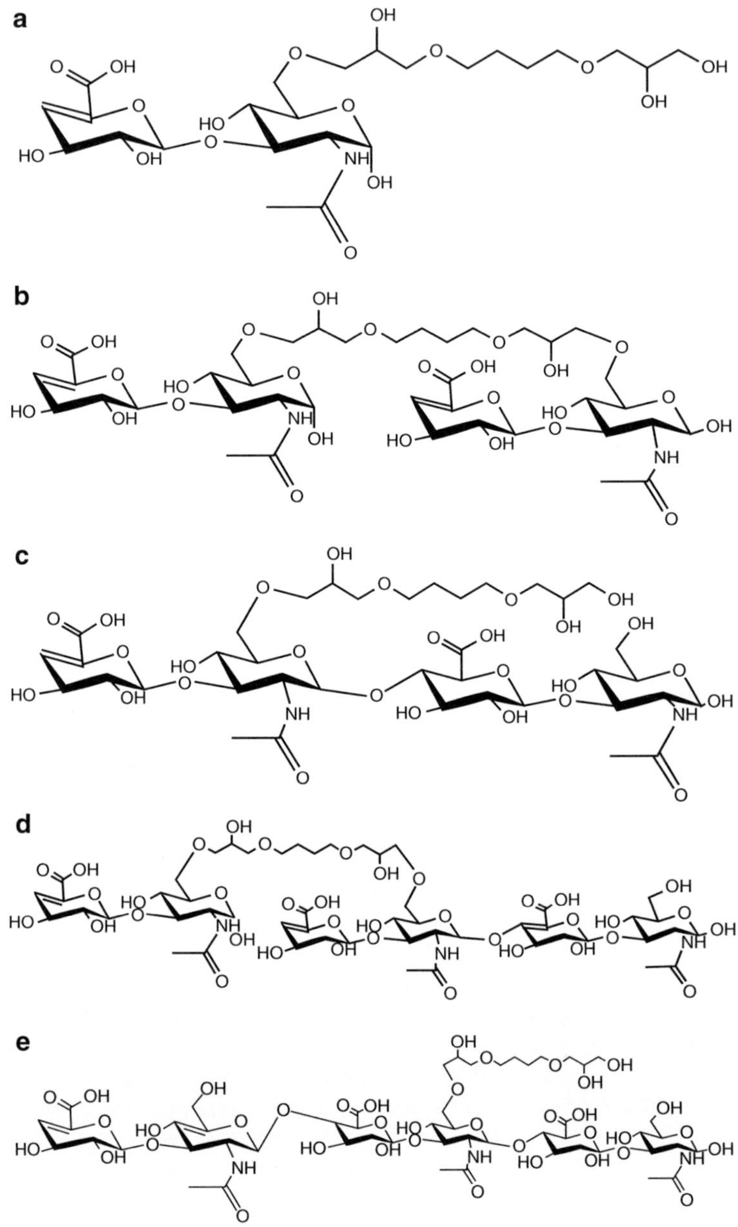

Fig. 5.5 Multiple structures of HA filler after degradation by chondroitinase. (**a**) HA and pendant BDPE. (**b**) Two HA and proper crosslinked BDPE. (**c**) Two HA and one pendant BDPE. (**d**) Three HA with two proper crosslinked BDPE. (**e**) Three HA with one pendant BDPE

liquid helium and liquid nitrogen, allowing for simple results to be obtained. However, due to the weak magnetic field, the sensitivity is generally low. ^{1}H (proton) data is possible, while ^{13}C data is not favorable.

The principle of NMR (shown in Fig. 5.6) involves atomic nuclei containing carbon or hydrogen, which carry a positive charge (atomic nuclei consist of protons (charge) and neutrons (mass), both of which spin around their axes, known as the nuclear spin). When they spin, they act similar to magnets. Light amplification by stimulated emission radiation (LASER) machines are well-known devices in aesthetic

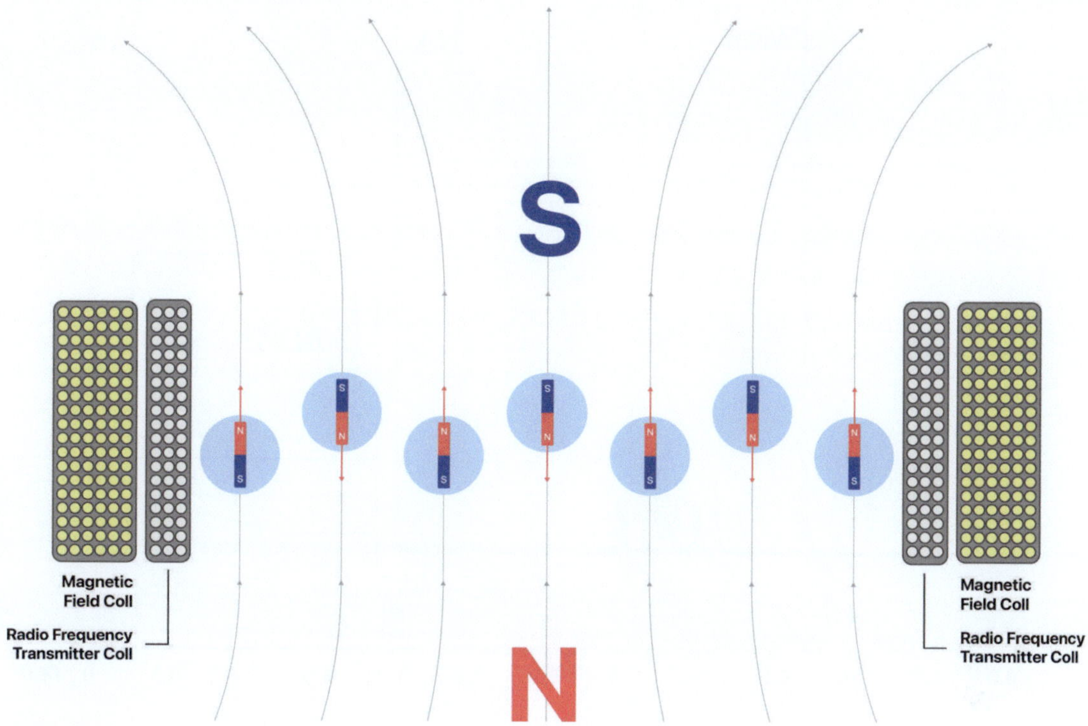

Fig. 5.6 Principle of NMR

medicine and LASER usually uses electron for energy. Electrons are known for spin movement, but atoms also have a spin, which is utilized in NMR devices. Nuclei spin freely, but when an external magnetic field is applied, they align in a parallel manner (either in the same direction or in the opposite direction as the magnetic field). When aligned in a parallel manner, they absorb energy (i.e., radio waves). When electromagnetic radiation occurs, spin flip occurs, and at this point, the atomic nuclei are said to resonate with the electromagnetic radiation. In other words, the excited state of the atomic nuclei, which absorbs energy from electromagnetic waves, returns to the ground state and emits energy. By detecting the electromagnetic waves emitted from these atomic nuclei and processing them appropriately, the results appear in the form of a spectrum. It is necessary to measure the energy generated by spinning atoms in a row, as it varies depending on the surrounding electron density, and this is measured as a frequency.

5.4 NMR Analysis: Spectrum Analysis

^{1}H NMR is a widely used technique, and the phenomenon is attributed to the electrons surrounding ^{1}H. The term "chemical shift" is used based on TMS (tetramethylsilane, silicon, 0 ppm), and is measured in terms of δ or ppm (0–10 ppm). Whenever NMR analysis is performed, silicon is added, and the peak appearing from TMS is taken as the 0 ppm reference. However, the peak values resulting from the chemical shift are referred to as chemical equivalence when they are in equivalent environments according to the chemical structure. In the case of HA filler, when viewed with reference to hydrogen, peak values appear at 1.5 and 2.0 (Fig. 5.7).

However, the combined structure of HA and BDDE is a more complex molecule; therefore, the ^{13}C results may be more accurate than the ^{1}H results. Thirteen commercially available HA fillers were evaluated by ^{1}H and ^{13}C NMR analysis (Fig. 5.8).

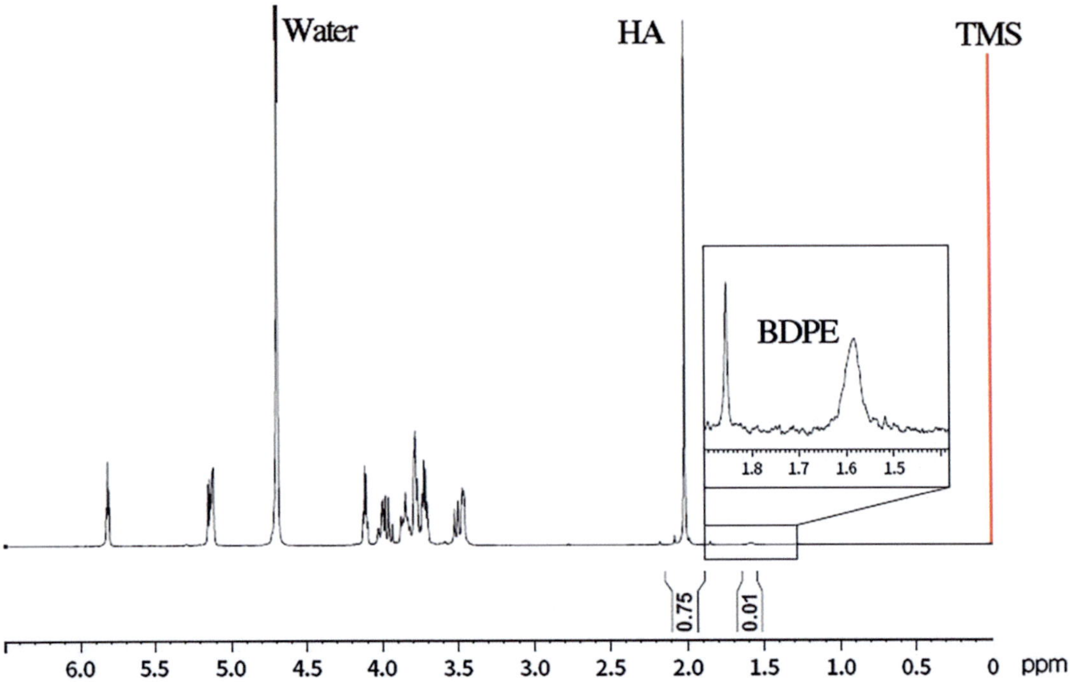

Fig. 5.7 Hyaluronic acid filler and BDPE NMR

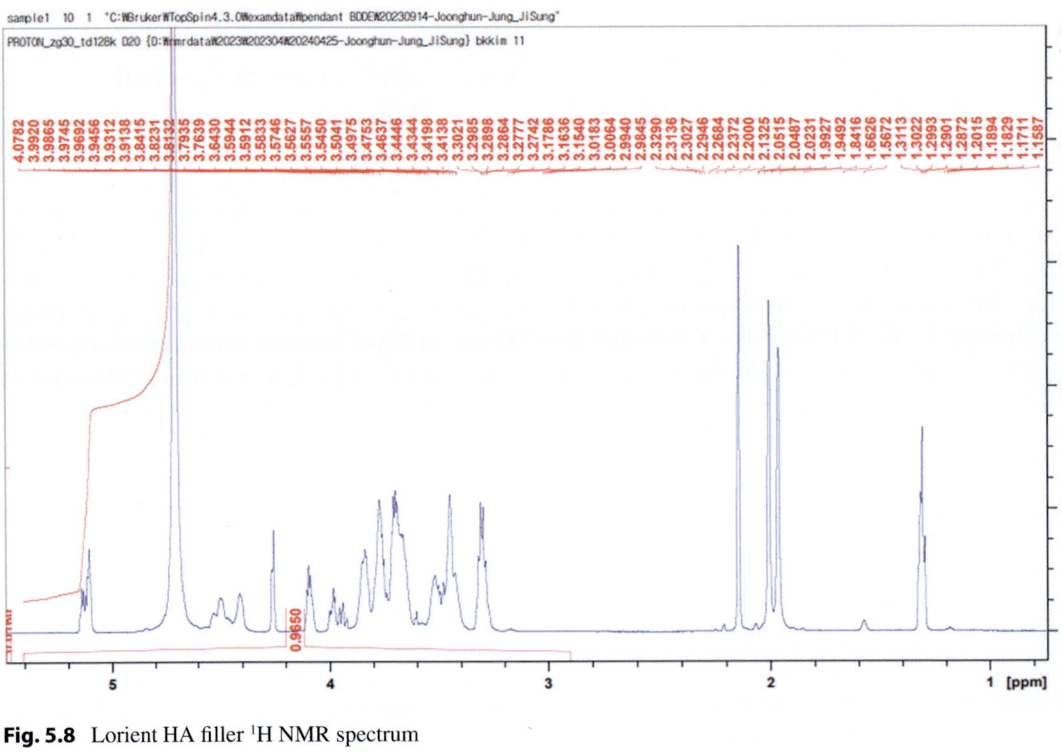

Fig. 5.8 Lorient HA filler ^{1}H NMR spectrum

5.5 Hyaluronic Acid Filler NMR Analysis Preparation

First, 13 HA fillers are selected to prepare the samples for NMR measurements. One gram of each filler is placed in a phosphate buffer solution and mixed with 100 U of chondroitinase ABC. The mixture was shaken for 48 h to dissolve. After freeze-drying, D_2O solution is added to a 5 mL NMR tube and placed in the NMR machine. For ^{13}C measurements, one feed was measured for 26 h (Fig. 5.9). The overall experimental process is shown in the figure (Fig. 5.10).

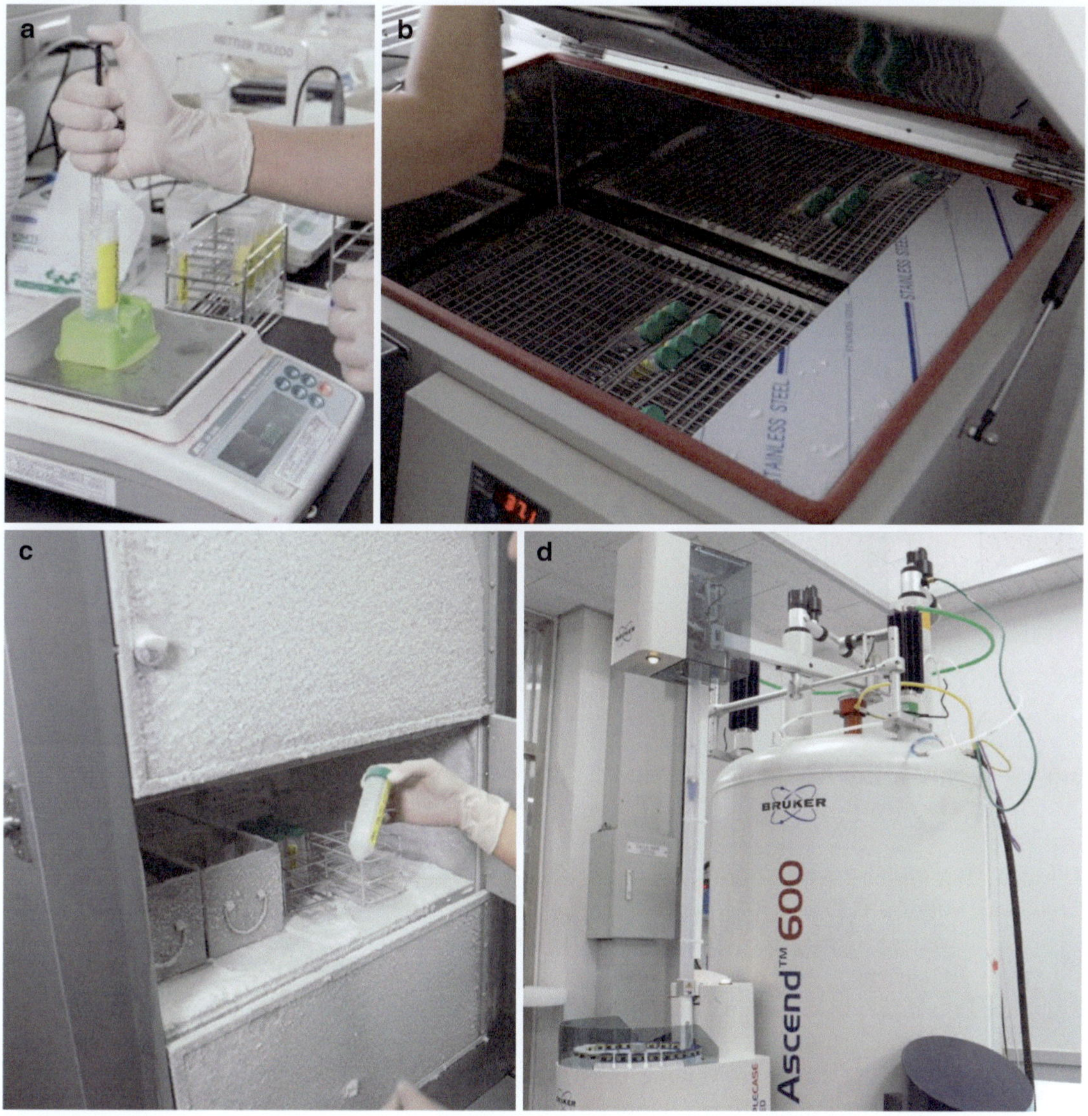

Fig. 5.9 NMR preparation. (**a**) Phosphate buffer solution and mixed with 100 U of chondroitinase. (**b**) React for 48 h. (**c**) Freeze-drying. (**d**) NMR test

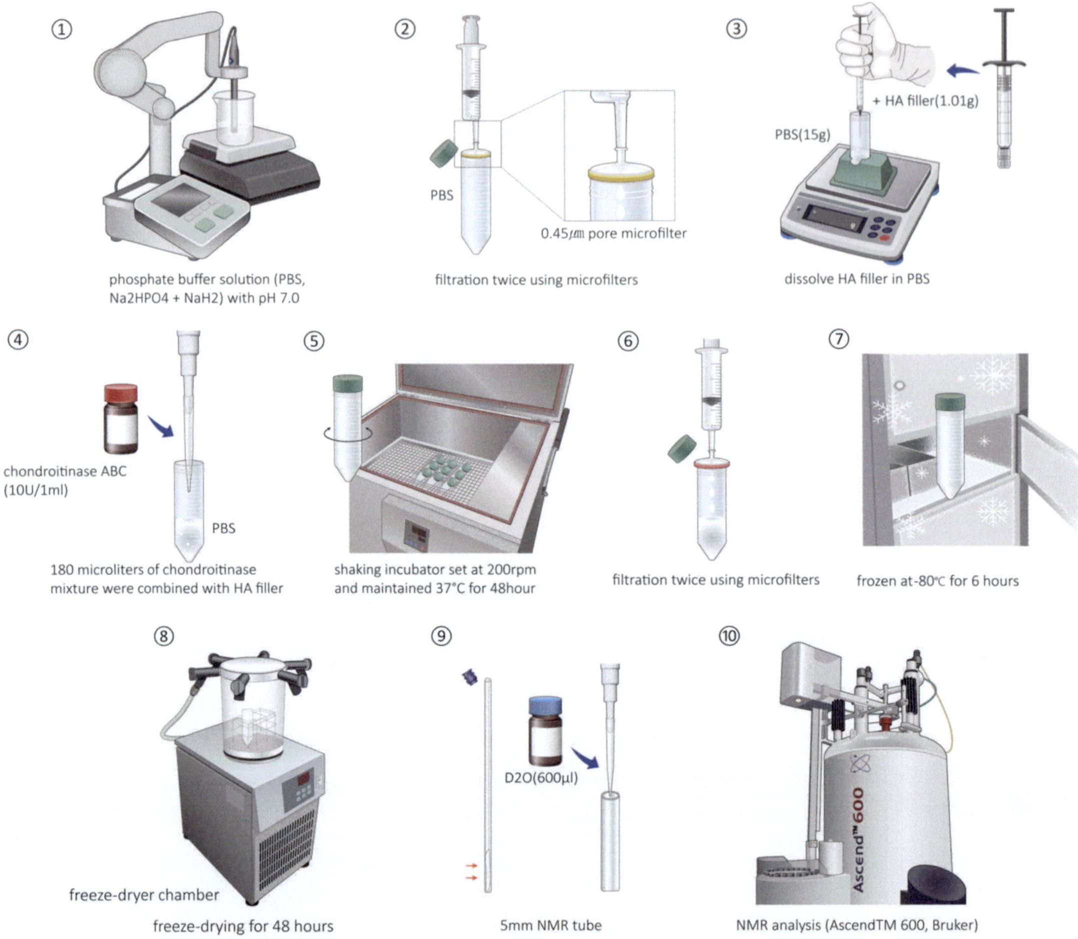

Fig. 5.10 NMR sample preparation and test

5.6 Hyaluronic Acid Filler Used at the Test

Thirteen HA fillers were used for testing. Restylane Volyme (LOT: 17031-1, Galderma, Uppsala, Sweden), Restylane Defyne (LOT: 18681-1, Galderma, Uppsala, Sweden), Restylane Lyft (LOT: 19765, Galderma, Uppsala, Sweden), Juvederm Voluma (LOT: 1000561748, Allergan, Irvine, CA), Belotero Volume (LOT: B00016110, Merz Pharmaceuticals, Frankfurt, Germany), Teosyal RHA4 (LOT: 22372DL03128, TEOXANE Laboratories, Geneva, Switzerland), L'orient No. 6 (LOT: J21001, Joonghun Pharmaceutical, Seoul, Republic of Korea), Neuramis Volume (LOT C523010A, Medy-Tox, Seoul, Republic of Korea), The Chaeum Premium No. 4 (LOT: BLD21008, HUGEL, Seoul, Republic of Korea), Elravie Deep (LOT: D6016002AA, Humedix, Seoul, Republic of Korea), Eptq S500 (LOT YLC22006, Jetema, Seoul, Republic of Korea), QTfill SubQ (LOT: QPAI21001G, S.THEPHARM, Seoul, Republic of Korea), and Youthfill Shape (LOT: YDE19013, RFBio, Seoul, Republic of Korea).

5.6.1 Mod, CrR, CrD

Thereon, we measured the amount of BDPE contained in the HA filler, which was measured as the modification of degree (MoD). In other words, the extent to which the original HA was modified by the attachment of BDDE. However, as mentioned previously, not all BDPE are properly attached; therefore, the number of pendants is also important. The crosslinked ratio (CrR) is one such measure, which is the ratio of properly attached crosslinkers to those that are already attached. In addition, the degree of crosslinking (CrD) is the product of MoD and CrR. These three parameters have been described in previous literature [3]. Their equations are as follows:

1. MoD (%, ^{1}H) = $(I^{\delta H1.6}/4)/(I^{\delta H2.0}/3) \times 100$
2. MoD (%, ^{13}C) = $(I^{\delta c25.2}/2)/I^{\delta c1.9\text{–}22.6} \times 100$
3. CrR = $1 - I^{\delta C62.7}/(I^{\delta 25.2}/2)$
4. CrD (%) = (CrR × MoD) × 100

The ^{1}H NMR value was obtained using 32 scans, and the ^{13}C NMR value was obtained after 4096 scans. The numerical values appearing in the spectra were calculated using MoD (%, ^{1}H) = $(I^{\delta H1.6}/4)/(I^{\delta H2.0}/3) \times 100$, i.e., using the values shifted at 1.6 and 2.0. For MoD (%, ^{13}C) = $(I^{\delta c25.2}/2)/I^{\delta c1.9\text{–}22.6} \times 100$, CrR = $1 - I^{\delta C62.7}/(I^{\delta c25.2}/2)$ were used for quantification. The values analyzed for the 13 fillers are listed in Table 5.1.

Structurally, this can be compared by examining the extent to which BDPE is typically attached to a hundred monomers of HA. A diagram of all the fillers used in the experiment is shown in Fig. 5.11. A graphical comparison of Lorient filler and HA filler product 5 is also depicted (Fig. 5.12).

When the biphasic filler method was used, the amount of BDDE decreases and MoD becomes lower. However, when using the monophasic filler method, naturally, a larger amount of BDDE must be added to achieve a certain predictable rheological data via crosslinking. However, there is no precise study on how our bodies react to the addition of a large amount of a crosslinking agent, but a high level of crosslinking agent makes it relatively more likely for our bodies' immune system to detect foreign substance. Above all, the CrR value is most important. For sample 5 HA filler, the MoD value is approximately 12–17%, but the CrR is 0.086. This indicates that although a large amount of BDDE was added during the manufacturing process, the actual amount of properly attached BDPE was minimal.

However, this is not necessarily the sole cause of delayed inflammatory reactions. As described in Chap. 6, foreign substances such as Si, Al, and other metals contained in HA fillers could be one cause, or it could be due to the molecular weight of HA. However, it is clear that fillers with minimal crosslinking and minimal pendant BDPE, as well as minimal foreign substances, are the cleanest HA fillers. It is natural for the cleanest fillers to cause the least amount of adverse effects.

Table 5.1 MoD and CrR analysis for 13 HA products

Product	MoD (%, ^{1}H)	MoD (%, ^{13}C)	CrR (^{13}C)	CrD (%, ^{13}C)	NMR reading date
1 A	11.215	8.187	0.394	3.232	20230724
2 B	10.194	9.723	0.085	0.824	20230425
3 C	2.370	2.112	0.117	0.246	20230918
4 D	8.789	7.103	0.143	1.015	20230819
5 E	17.065	12.567	0.086	1.077	20230803
6 F	6.303	4.915	0.118	0.581	20230807
7 Lorient	2.239	1.947	0.227	0.443	20230914
8 H	14.748	9.904	0.014	0.204	20230804
9 I	14.476	12.101	0.333	4.034	20230728
10 J	10.912	9.269	0.141	1.304	20230726
11 K	4.748	2.999	0.049	0.146	20230725
12 L	8.055	4.747	0.065	0.306	20230731
13 M	7.192	6.147	0.343	2.110	20230820

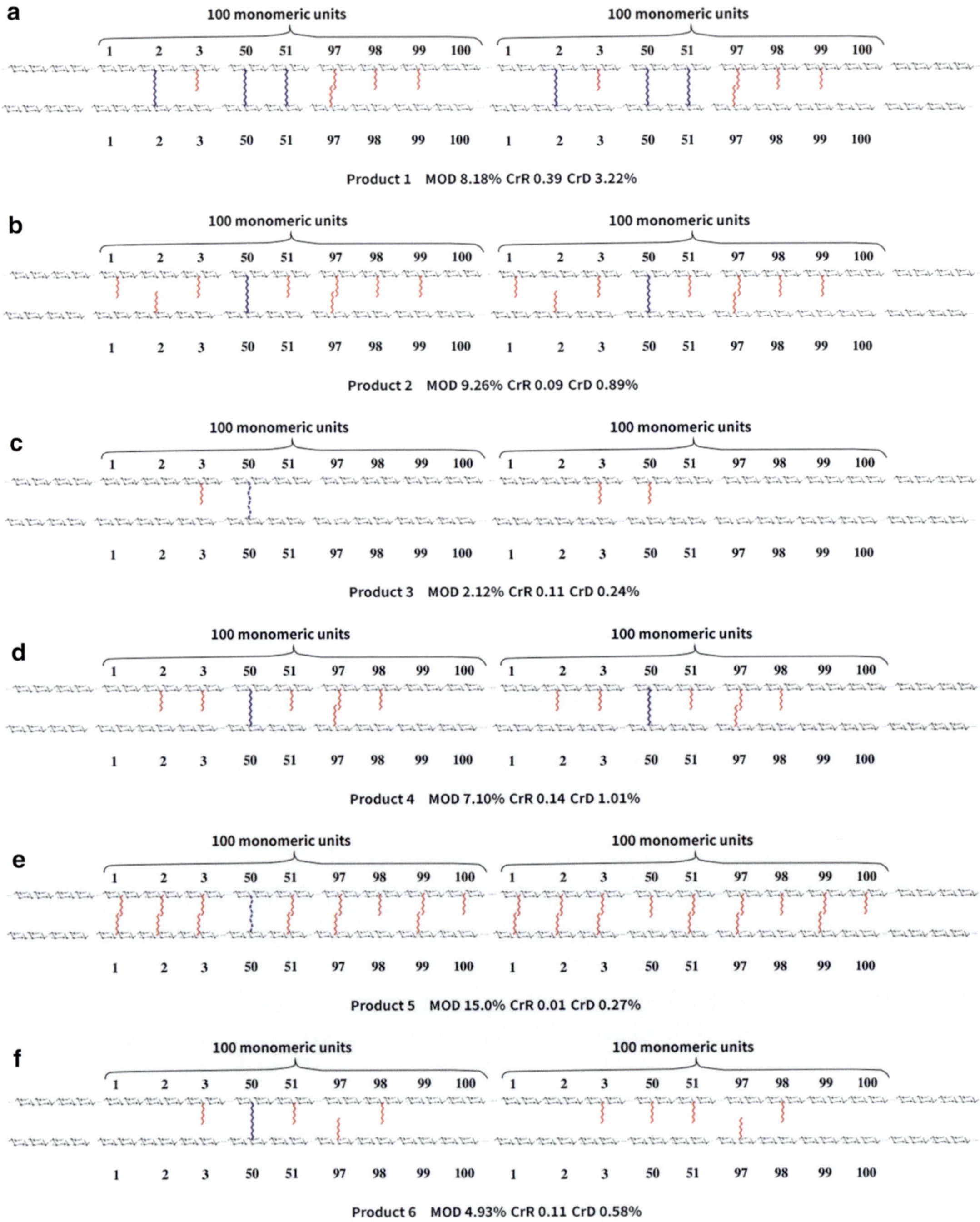

Fig. 5.11 Schematic diagram of HA fillers

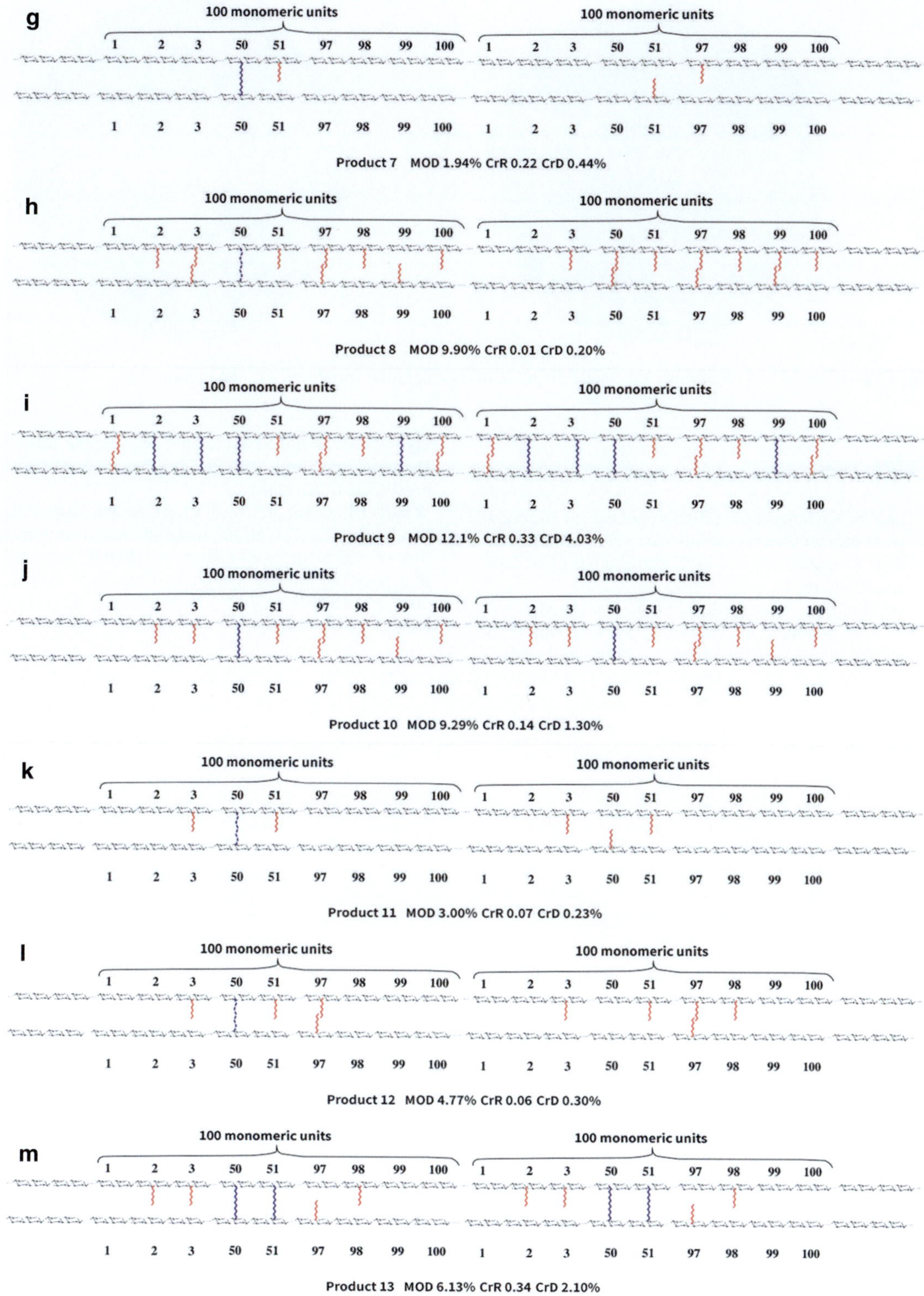

Fig. 5.11 (continued)

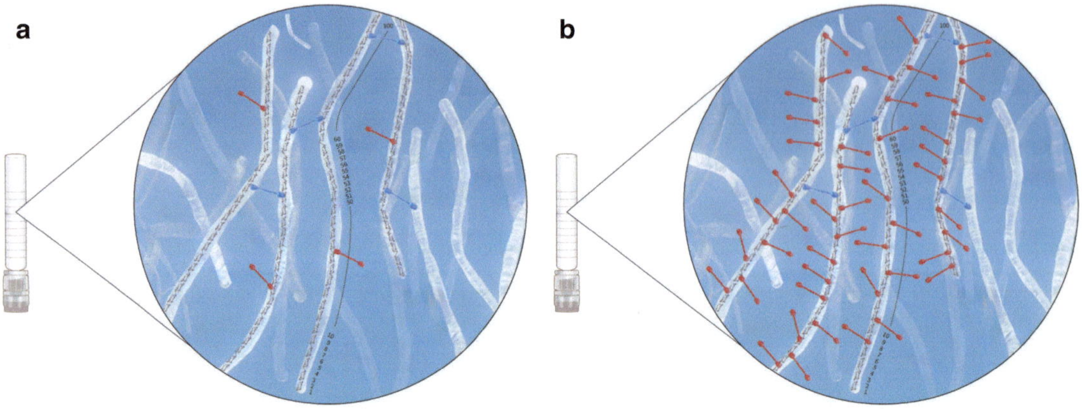

Fig. 5.12 HA filler and crosslinker schematic diagram. (**a**) Lorient filler (product 7 G). (**b**) Product 5 E

References

1. Lee W. Comments on “Hyaluronidase: an overview of its properties, applications, and side effects”. Arch Plast Surg. 2020;47(6):626–7. https://doi.org/10.5999/aps.2020.01571.
2. De Boulle K, Glogau R, Kono T, Nathan M, Tezel A, Roca-Martinez JX, Paliwal S, Stroumpoulis D. A review of the metabolism of 1,4-butanediol diglycidyl ether-crosslinked hyaluronic acid dermal fillers. Dermatologic Surg. 2013;39(12):1758–66. https://doi.org/10.1111/dsu.12301.
3. Wende FJ, Gohil S, Nord LI, Helander Kenne A, Sandström C. 1D NMR methods for determination of degree of cross-linking and BDDE substitution positions in HA hydrogels. Carbohydr Polym. 2017;157:1525–30. https://doi.org/10.1016/j.carbpol.2016.11.029.

6 Hyaluronic Acid Filler Impurities

Contents

6.1 Introduction

Generally, hyaluronic acid (HA) is distributed in a powdered form and is divided into several grades based on its purity and other factors. Typically, 1,4-butanediol diglycidyl (BDDE) is used as a crosslinking agent in addition to other substances such as polyethylene glycol (PEG) or divinylsulfone (DVS). The addition of powdered HA and a crosslinking agent results in the formation of HA fillers, and the manufacturing process involves several other steps.

HA fillers should theoretically consist only of HA and a crosslinking agent. During these manufacturing processes, impurities are introduced and in order to obtain purer fillers, these impurities should be minimized. In this chapter, we explore the manufacturing process of HA fillers and describe the impurities that arise, as well as how they may impact delayed swelling.

6.2 Manufacturing Process

Understanding the manufacturing process of HA fillers allows for an understanding of the rheological properties of the filler and where impurities may arise.

As described above, HA is available in powder form. When it reacts with a crosslinking

W. Lee, *Advances in Hyaluronic Acid Filler Injections*,
https://doi.org/10.1007/978-981-97-6528-7_6

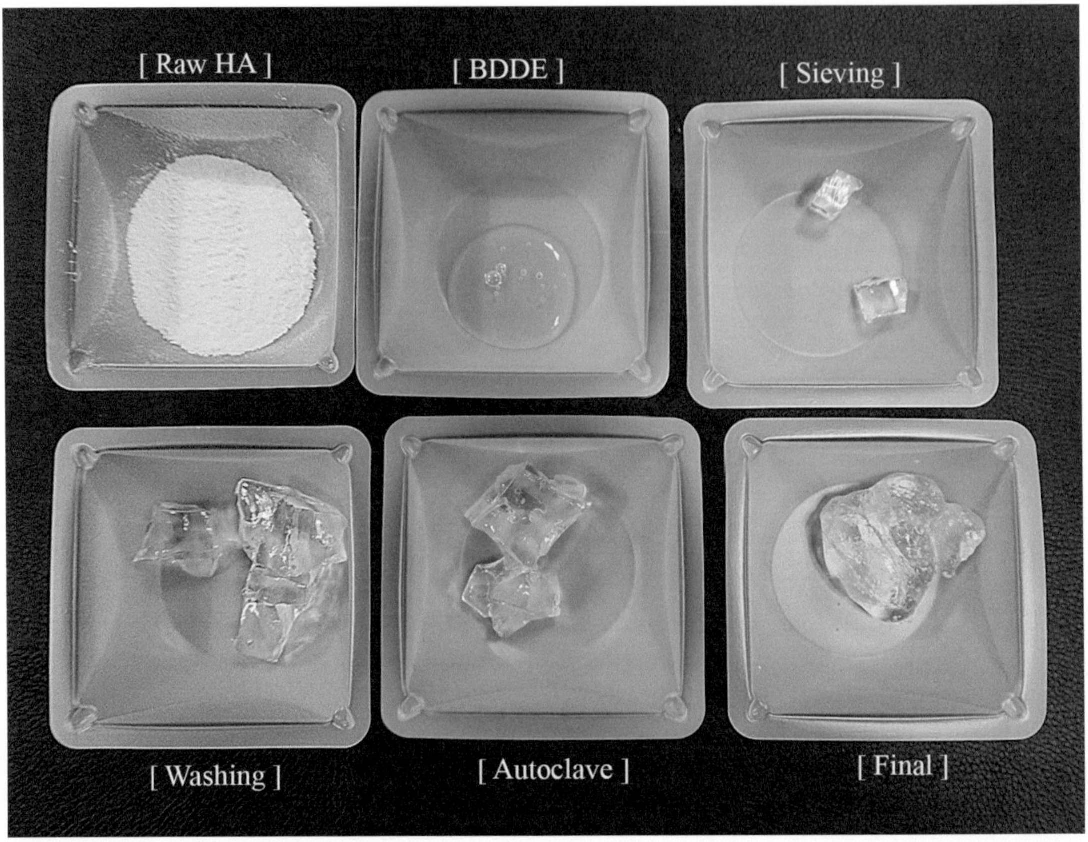

Fig. 6.1 HA filler change during the manufacturing process

agent, it becomes a liquid, which is then transformed into the HA filler used in various processes (Fig. 6.1). We now consider the manufacturing process in more detail.

Reaction, washing, and sterilization are essential steps in the production of HA, while other dialysis processes may vary slightly from manufacturer to manufacturer (Fig. 6.2). The reaction process involves mixing HA with a crosslinking agent and reacting BDDE with a strong base to induce crosslinking, sometimes using a strong acid. Therefore, the cleaning process must be thorough to remove impurities. In addition, impurities may be generated if the reaction is performed in aluminum vats. Finally, the HA filler is placed in a syringe and sterilized at 121 °C, which could also have some impurities. Figure 6.3 is an outline of the process. Impurities may be present in the water used to produce the HA filler and in the raw HA material. In addition, as mentioned above, impurities may occur during the reaction process, such as dissolution with NaOH, and may appear in the manufacturing chamber or grinder. Last but not least, impurities may also arise from the syringe.

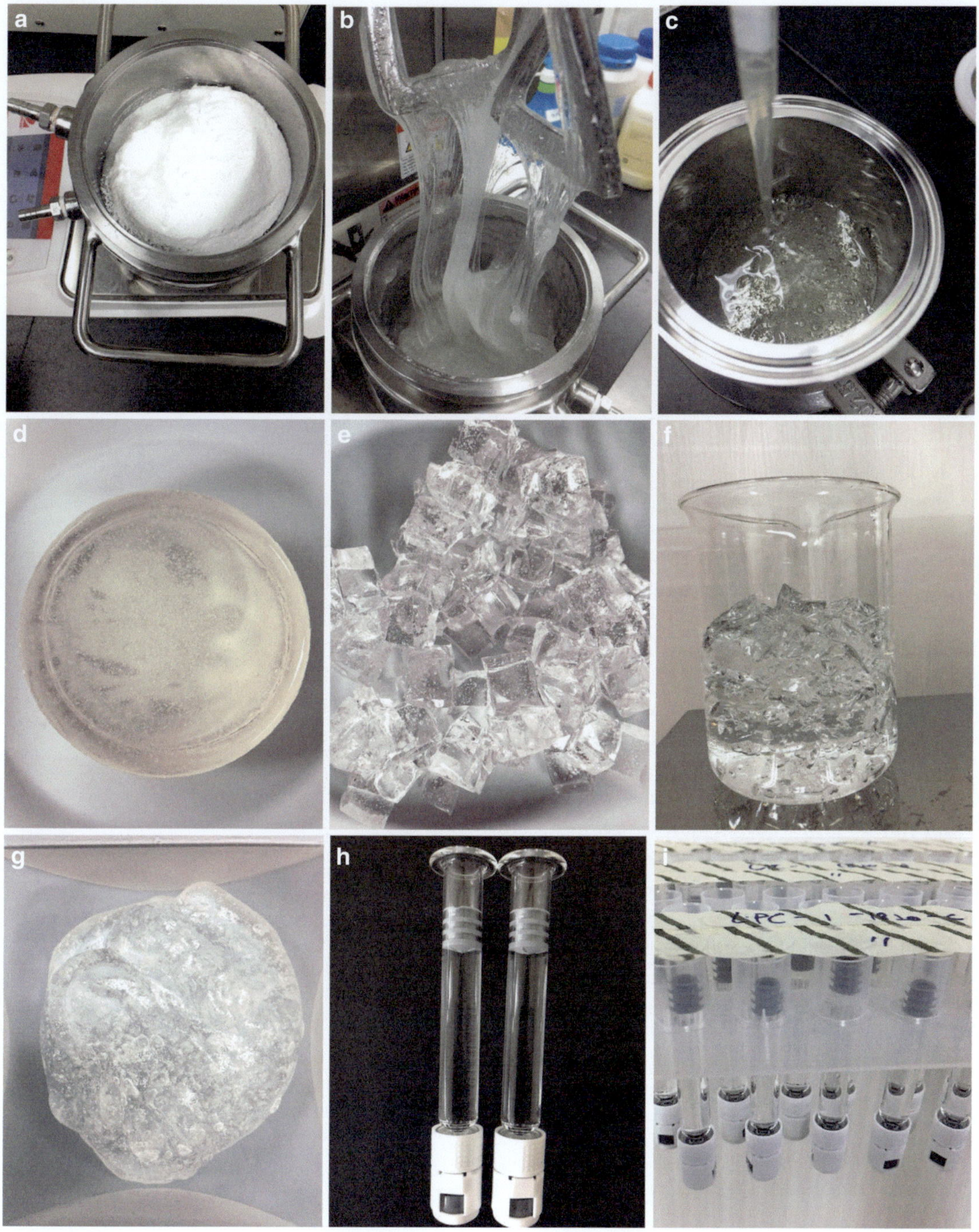

Fig. 6.2 Hyaluronic acid filler manufacturing process. (**a**) Weight: Weigh raw hyaluronic acid. (**b**) Dissolve in NaOH. (**c**) Reaction: Mix with 1,4 butanediol diglycidyl ether at appropriate times and temperatures. (**d**) Gel after reaction. (**e**) Cutting: Cut the gel to appropriate size. (**f**) Washing: Wash-off remaining NaOH, free 1,4 butanediol diglycidyl ether, and hyaluronic impurities. (**g**) Sieving: Sieve for the appropriate size. (**h**) Filling: Fill the syringe. (**i**) Autoclave

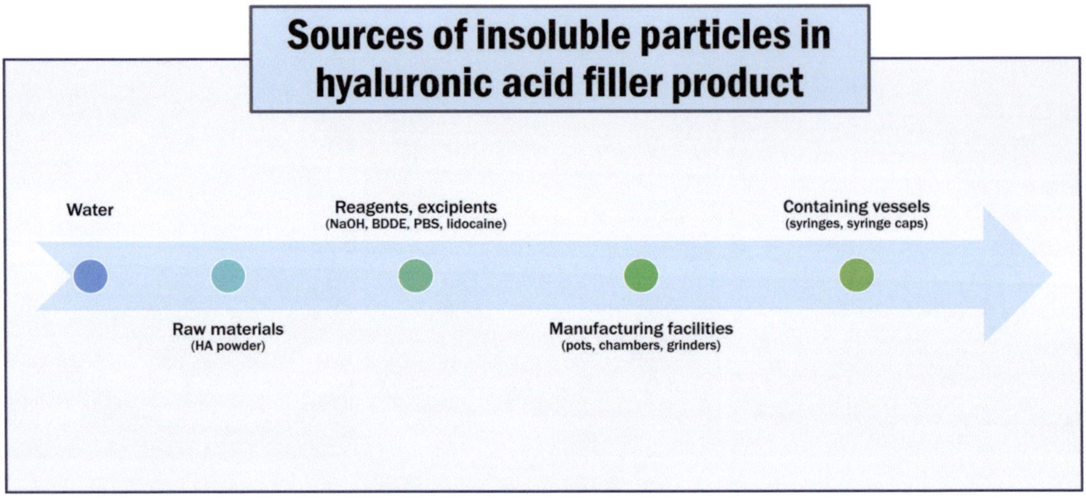

Fig. 6.3 Sources of HA filler impurities during manufacturing process

6.3 Impurities During Manufacturing Process

Generally, pharmaceuticals contain impurities. Even if the product is very clean, a small amount of impurities can still be present, as mentioned by the US Food and Drug Administration (FDA) [1]. Various impurities can be present, including silicon, metals, proteins, and dust (Table 6.1). However, in many cases, these impurities can cause various side effects; thus, permissible limits have been established. These particles are classified as visible particles (>100 μm) and subvisible particles, and specific limits have been set for the subvisible particles that are not visible to the naked eye. Both the FDA [2] and the European Directorate for the Quality of Medicines & HealthCare (EDQM) [3] have established criteria for the number of particles allowed in a single prefilled syringe, with limits of 600 or fewer particles larger than 25 μm and 6000 or fewer particles larger than 10 μm.

Table 6.1 Particles in syringe

Type	Source	Example
Extrinsic	Contamination from an external source	Dust Particles of biological origin
Intrinsic	Particles derived from contact of the product with materials used in the containers or packaging	Silicone particles Polymeric materials Metal particles Glass particles Rubber particles
Inherent	Particles related to the process – The result of interactions with the manufacturing equipment during the production process – May arise from physical or chemical changes during the production process	Protein aggregates Colloidal formulations Insoluble degradation products' active ingredients Crystals of active ingredients Metal particles

6.4 Hyaluronic Acid Filler Impurities

However, the standards for foreign substances are not applicable to HA fillers. HA fillers are classified as medical devices rather than injectable agents; therefore, they are not subject to the standards applied to injectable agents. However, HA fillers can enter the human body. Moreover, many foreign substances can trigger immune responses and cause delayed inflammatory swelling. Therefore, we measured the number of particles inside the HA fillers. A total of 12 HA fillers were measured (Fig. 6.4).

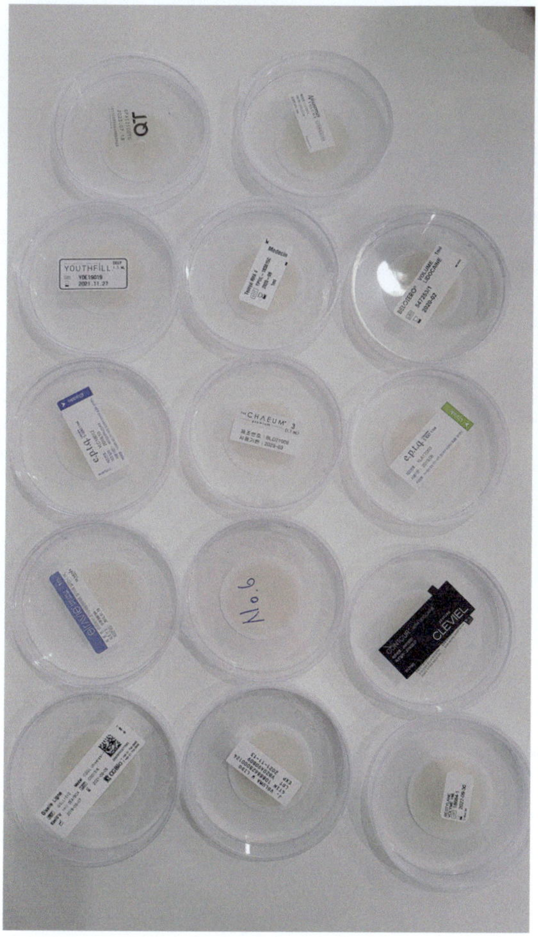

Fig. 6.4 HA filler impurities test samples

Restylane Volume (LOT 18684-1, Galderma, Uppsala, Sweden), Juvéderm Voluma (LOT VB20A90809, Allergan, Irvine, CA, USA), Belotero Volume (LOT 547253/1, Merz Pharmaceuticals, Frankfurt, Germany), Teosyal RHA4 (LOT TPUL-183815C, TEOXANE Laboratories, Geneva, Switzerland), L'orient No. 6 (LOT J20001, Joonghun Pharmaceutical, Seoul, Republic of Korea), Neuramis Volume (LOT C521007A, Medy-Tox, Seoul, Republic of Korea), The Chaeum Premium No. 3 (LOT BLD21008, HUGEL, Seoul, Republic of Korea), Elravie Deep (LOT D1915001BA, Humedix, Seoul, Republic of Korea), Eptq S500 (LOT YLC18012, Jetema, Seoul, Republic of Korea), QTfill SubQ (QPAI21001G, S.THEPHARM, Seoul, Republic of Korea), Youthfill Deep (LOT YDE19019, RFBio, Seoul, Republic of Korea), and Cleviel Contour (LOT J94118001, PharmaResearch, Seongnam, Republic of Korea).

6.5 Experimental Methods

The experimental method is illustrated (Fig. 6.5). First, the HA filler is dissolved in hyaluronidase. The mixture is then completely dissolved in a shaking tank for 24 h. The particle count is then measured three times using an insoluble particle counter (Fig. 6.6). The sample is then placed on a filter paper and observed under an electron microscope to examine the shape of the particles. The electron microscope used for observation is a Quattro S SEM (Fig. 6.7). Subsequently, the composition of the visible particles was confirmed using energy-dispersive X-ray spectrometer analysis (EDS).

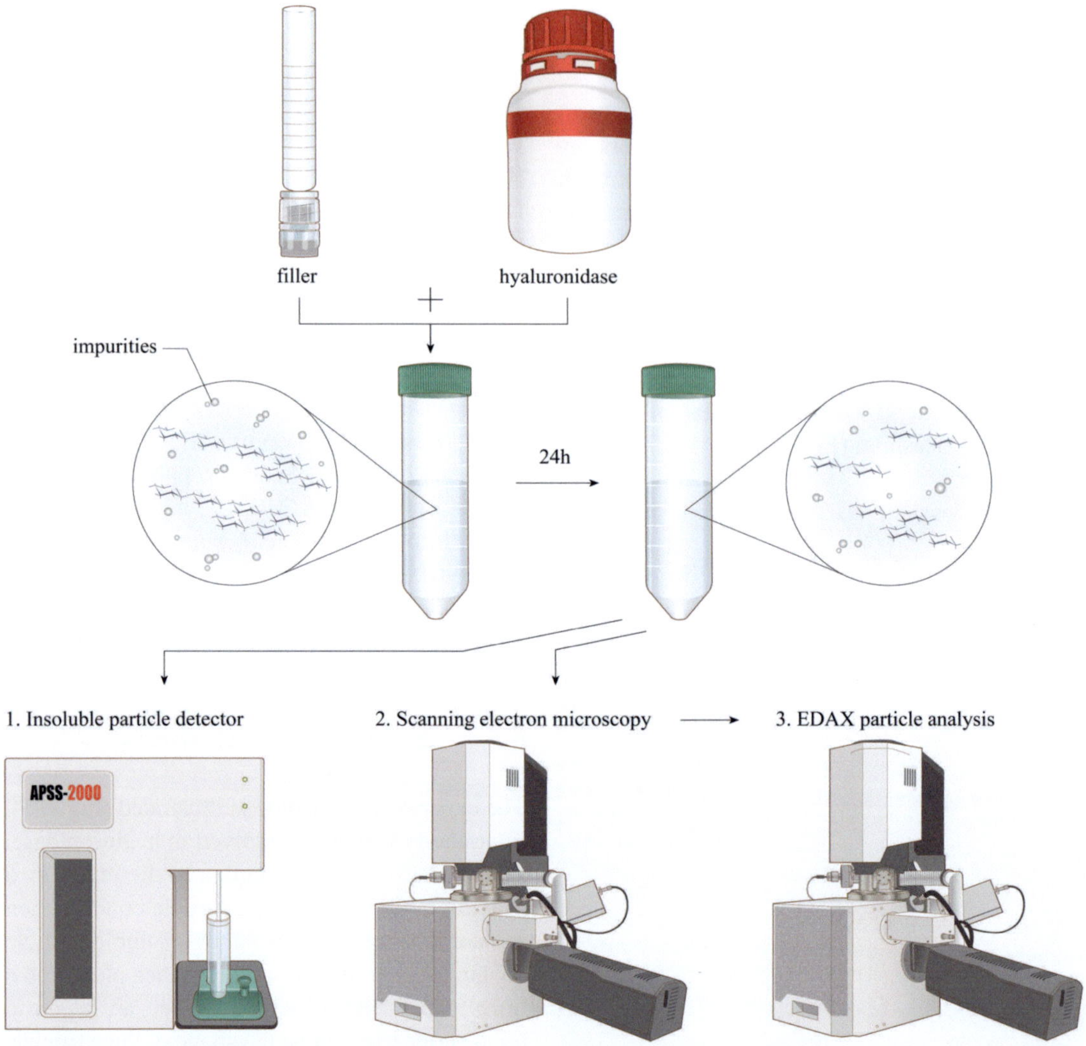

Fig. 6.5 Impurity particle analysis process

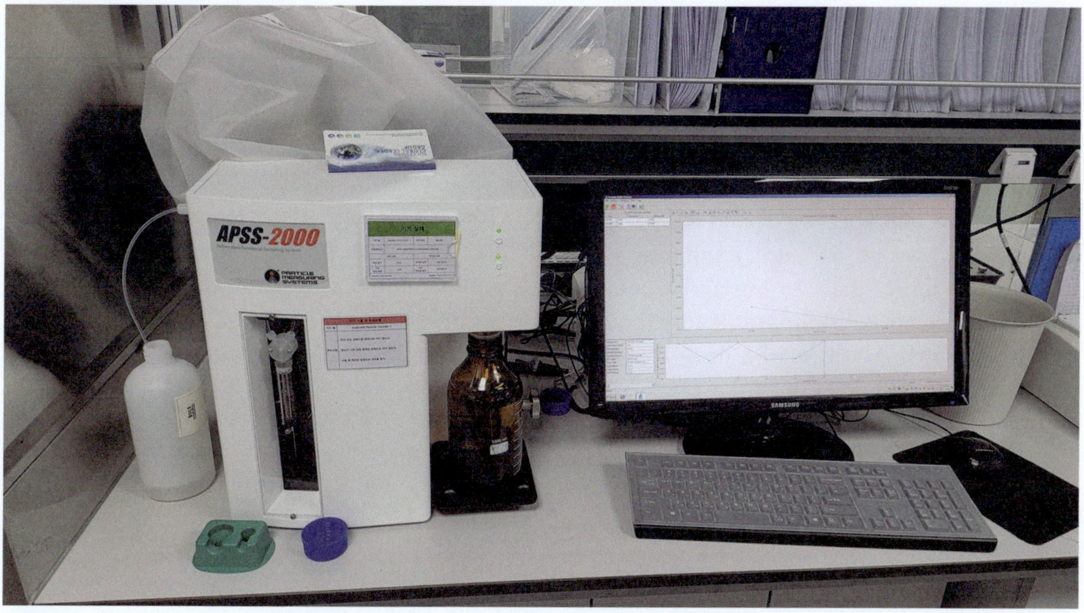

Fig. 6.6 Particle analyzer, APSS-2000 (Automated Parenteral Sampling System, Particle Measuring Systems, Boulder, CO, USA)

Fig. 6.7 Scanning electron microscope (2 °C, 747 Pa, 100% humidity, Quattro S SEM, approximately 250–5000×, Thermo Fisher, Waltham, MA, USA)

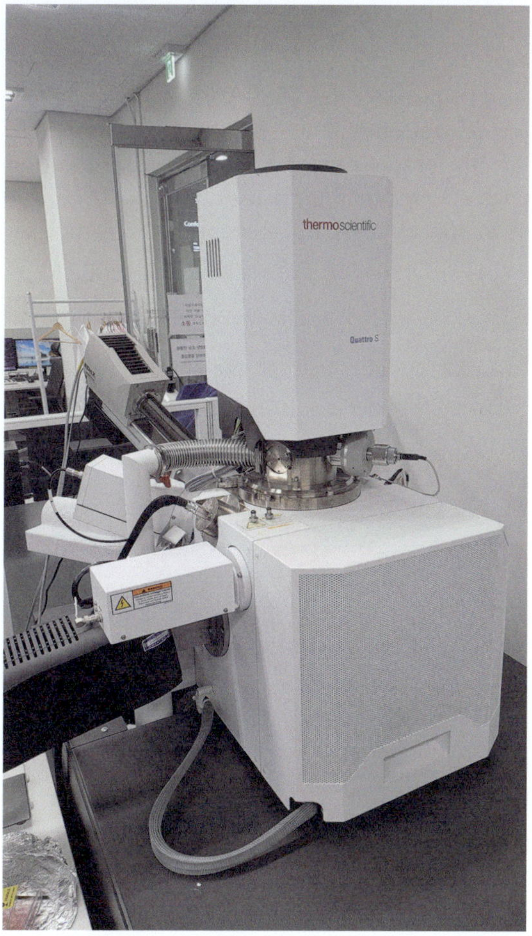

6.6 Results

6.6.1 Insoluble Particle Analysis

The particle counts are presented in Table 6.2.

After measuring each sample thrice and obtaining the average, we found seven fillers (A, B, C, D, Lorient, G, and J) suitable with a particle size larger than 25 µm and a count of 600 or less, as per the standards set by the FDA and the EDQM. Additionally, only five types of fillers (A, B, C, D, Lorient) were found to meet the criteria of having a particle size larger than 10 µm and a count of 6000 or less. In the case of HA filler I, the number of particles larger than 10 µm exceeded the allowable limit by approximately 20 times, with a count of 118,140. Furthermore, for particles with a size of 25 µm, the count was more than 10 times the allowable limit, at 6254.

6.6.2 SEM Analysis

As the presence of impurities was significant, scanning electron microscopy (SEM) was used to directly observe these impurities. The electron microscopic findings are as follows.

In the electron microscopic examination of Lorient filler, very few impurities were found (Fig. 6.8). The electron microscopic findings of the K filler were that the impurities of the same size were visible based on a 100 µm standard (Fig. 6.9). When magnified 1000 times, foreign substances with a size of 50 µm are clearly visible (Fig. 6.10).

Impurities were also clearly observed in the other HA fillers. In the case of Product G, at a magnification of 250×, multiple impurities were observed (Fig. 6.11).

In the case of J HA filler, impurities were also found, exhibiting a different appearance than the other products (Fig. 6.12). Additionally, in the case of Product L, impurities were discovered as slightly translucent foreign particles (Fig. 6.13).

6.6.3 EDS Analysis

After identifying impurities using SEM, the composition of these substances can be analyzed by focusing and passing X-rays through them. The composition table obtained using EDS is presented in Table 6.3.

The composition of the impurities can be analyzed when X-rays are passed through the HA fillers. In the case of the Lorient filler, C, O, and F were detected, corresponding to the values of the filter it contained (Fig. 6.14).

Table 6.2 HA filler products with variable counts of insoluble particles

	Larger than 10 µm (count/syringe)				Larger than 25 µm (count/syringe)			
	1st	2nd	3rd	Average	1st	2nd	3rd	Average
A	4048	3012	3528	3529	60	32	72	54
B	1352	1264	1272	1296	156	112	118	128
C	1304	968	828	1033	72	44	28	48
D	3632	3588	3536	3585	28	8	16	17
Lorient	1204	1340	1196	1246	88	72	88	82
F	76,520	79,792	76,588	77,633	812	1044	876	910
G	11,468	10,460	10,804	10,910	312	312	236	286
H	16,264	16,816	17,084	16,721	936	916	936	929
I	121,244	120,184	118,140	119,856	6156	6600	6008	6254
J	27,912	29,712	28,180	28,601	120	84	96	100
K	28,892	25,780	25,480	26,717	896	756	820	824
L	46,408	43,516	40,568	43,497	992	1100	1092	1061
Control	44	32	36	37	20	4	12	12

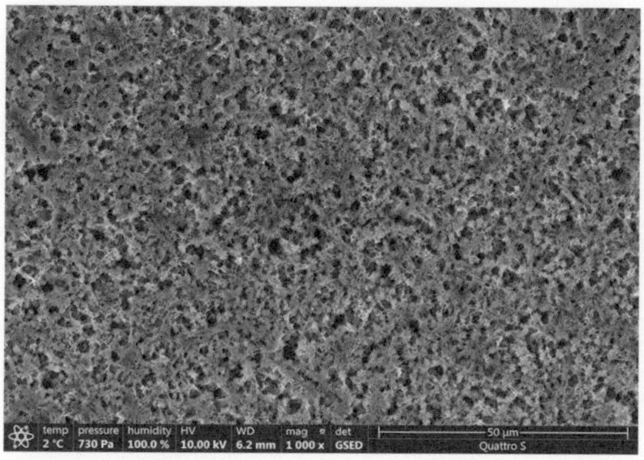

Fig. 6.8 Electron microscopic examination of Lorient filler. No impurities are visible, and only the filter appears as a sponge-like structure

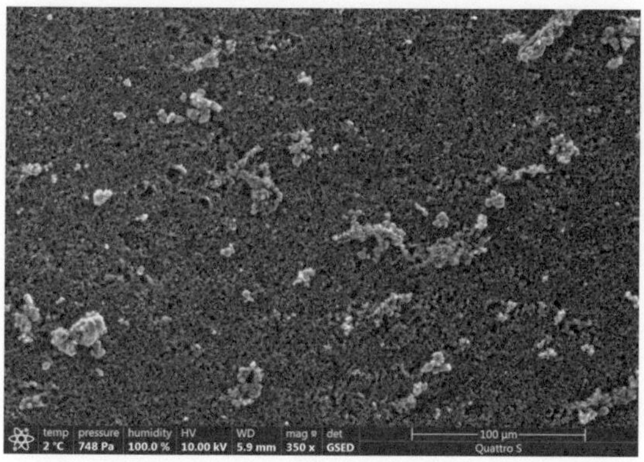

Fig. 6.9 Electron microscopic finding of the K filler (350×). 100 µm sized particles visible

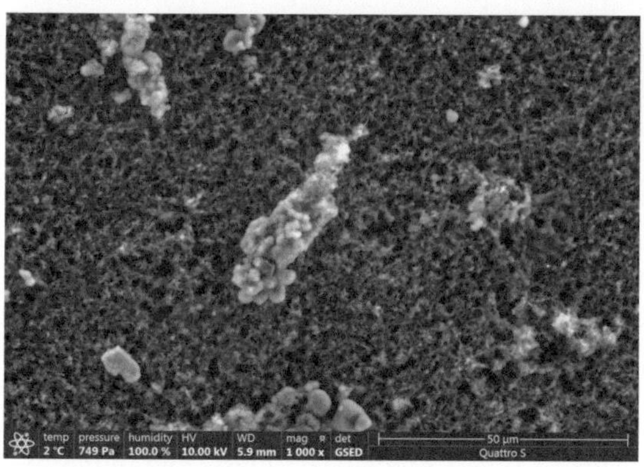

Fig. 6.10 Electron microscopic finding of K filler (1000×). 50 µm sized particles visible

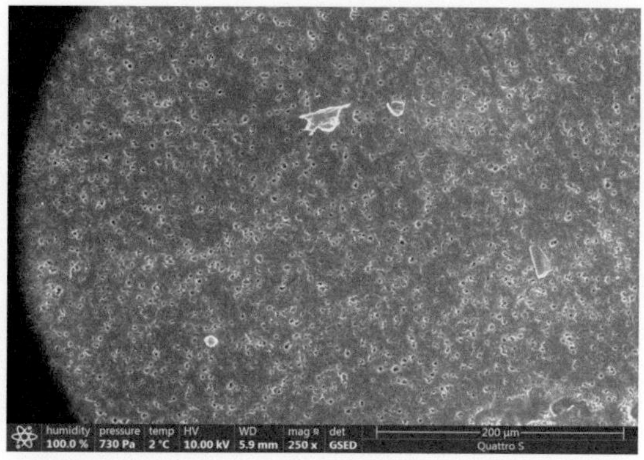

Fig. 6.11 Product G hyaluronic acid filler (250×)

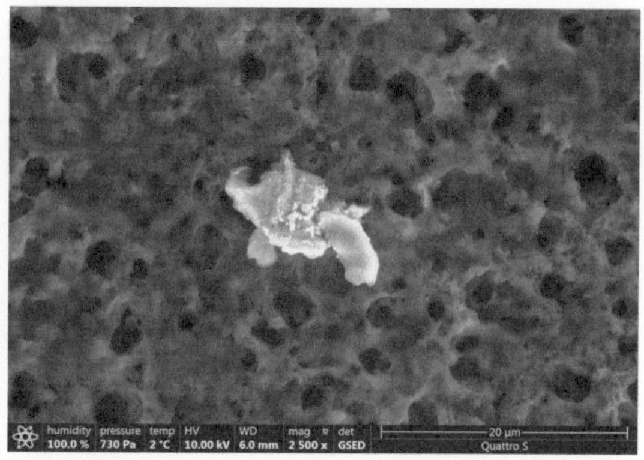

Fig. 6.12 Product J hyaluronic acid filler (2500×). 10 µm sized impurity visible

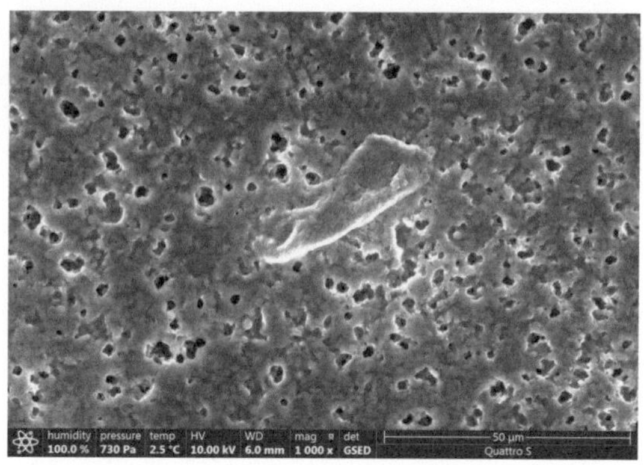

Fig. 6.13 Product L hyaluronic acid filler (1000×). 50 µm sized impurity visible

Table 6.3 EDS results

Filler product	SEM (particles detected)	EDS isotopes
A	Few	C O F Mg
B	Few	C O F Mg P
C	Very few	C O F Mg P
D	Few	C O F Mg Si P Ca
Lorient No. 6	Very few	C O F
F	Many	C O F Si Al Mg Ca
G	Few	C O F Si Al
H	Few	C O Si
I	Many	C O F Si Al P
J	Many	C O F Al Fe
K	Many	C O Si
L	Many	C O F Al Si P S Cl K Ca

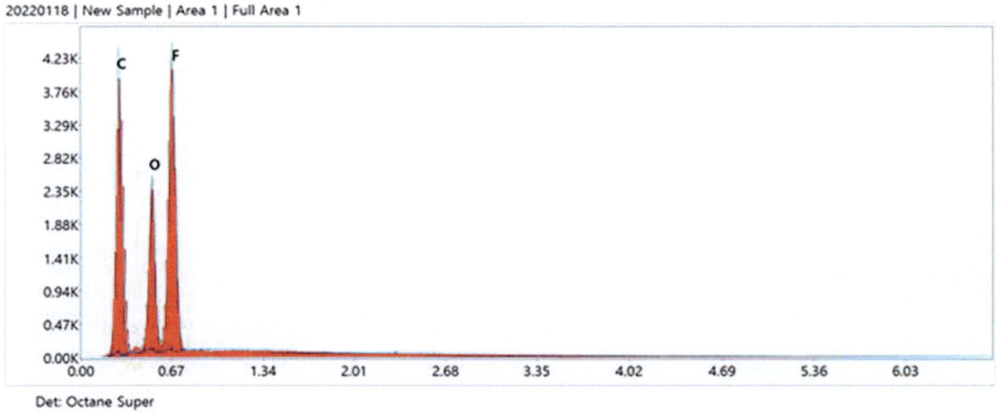

eZAF Quant Result - Analysis Uncertainty: 8.17 %

Element	Weight %	MDL	Atomic %	Net Int.	Error %	R	A	F
C K	53.2	0.33	62.4	823.0	7.7	0.9386	0.4772	1.0000
O K	21.3	0.26	18.8	521.6	9.1	0.9478	0.3787	1.0000
F K	25.5	0.17	18.9	960.1	8.3	0.9515	0.4320	1.0000

Fig. 6.14 EDS result of Lorient filler (atomic: mole ratio, Net Int.: real valid data, error %: error percentage <30% can be determined for data with confidence, A: absorbance, F: spectroscopy)

In contrast, the energy dispersive X-ray analysis (EDAX) analysis of the particles from Product G revealed the presence of silicone (Fig. 6.15). Silicone oil reportedly induces immunological tolerance and antibody responses [4]. Although silicone oil is commonly found in prefilled syringes for lubrication purposes, it can also form particles [5, 6]. Therefore, the detection of silicone may be a factor that could trigger immune reactions.

For the other product, J, aluminum was detected in the EDAX results (Fig. 6.16). The possible reason was that the prefilled syringe was made of type I borosilicate glass containing 5% aluminum oxide. The contaminant was also detected in the glass barrels and rubber stoppers during the filler manufacturing process [7, 8].

In addition, elements such as Ca and Mg were detected. These were detected in products D and F (Figs. 6.17 and 6.18). Generally, stainless steel

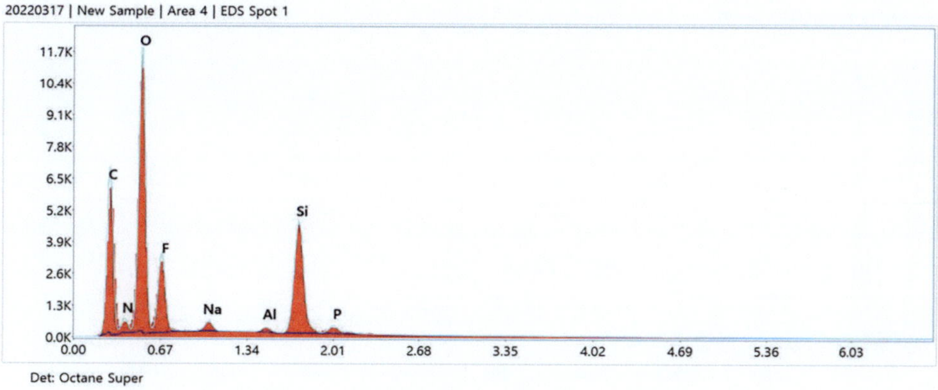

eZAF Quant Result - Analysis Uncertainty: 6.59 %

Element	Weight %	MDL	Atomic %	Net Int.	Error %	R	A	F
C K	39.9	0.22	48.6	1673.3	8.8	0.9347	0.3597	1.0000
N K	6.1	0.38	6.3	153.7	13.1	0.9401	0.2127	1.0000
O K	37.6	0.13	34.4	3194.1	8.6	0.9443	0.3662	1.0000
F K	8.6	0.11	6.6	910.5	9.6	0.9482	0.3388	1.0000
Na K	0.5	0.07	0.3	114.1	12.1	0.9552	0.6288	1.0024
Al K	0.2	0.05	0.1	65.3	12.3	0.9616	0.8364	1.0075
Si K	6.5	0.05	3.4	1700.6	3.8	0.9645	0.8921	1.0040
P K	0.5	0.07	0.3	114.3	8.6	0.9674	0.9085	1.0053

Fig. 6.15 EDAX result of product G. Silicone detected

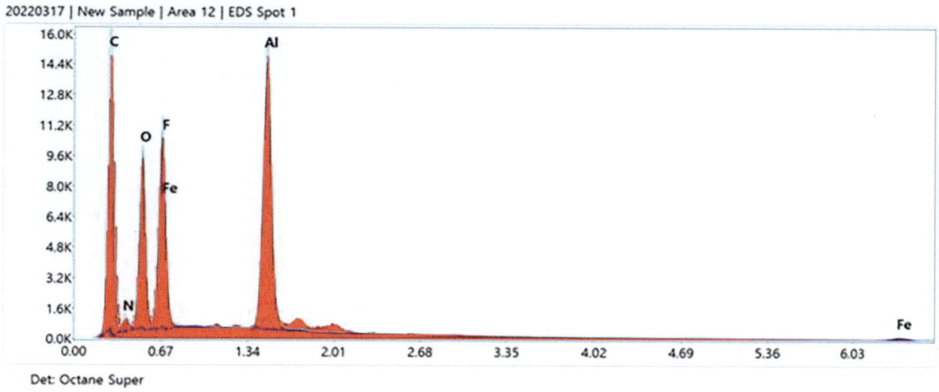

eZAF Quant Result - Analysis Uncertainty: 21.56 %

Element	Weight %	MDL	Atomic %	Net Int.	Error %	R	A	F
C K	50.6	0.18	61.6	3003.0	8.5	0.9322	0.3643	1.0000
N K	5.2	0.39	5.4	152.9	14.1	0.9377	0.1765	1.0000
O K	18.4	0.12	16.8	1959.3	9.1	0.9421	0.3276	1.0000
F K	12.9	0.08	10.0	2314.9	8.4	0.9461	0.4077	1.0000
Al K	9.9	0.04	5.3	3950.6	4.0	0.9600	0.8454	1.0026
Fe K	3.0	0.52	0.8	60.1	17.2	0.9935	0.9966	1.0898

Fig. 6.16 EDAX result of product J. Aluminum detected

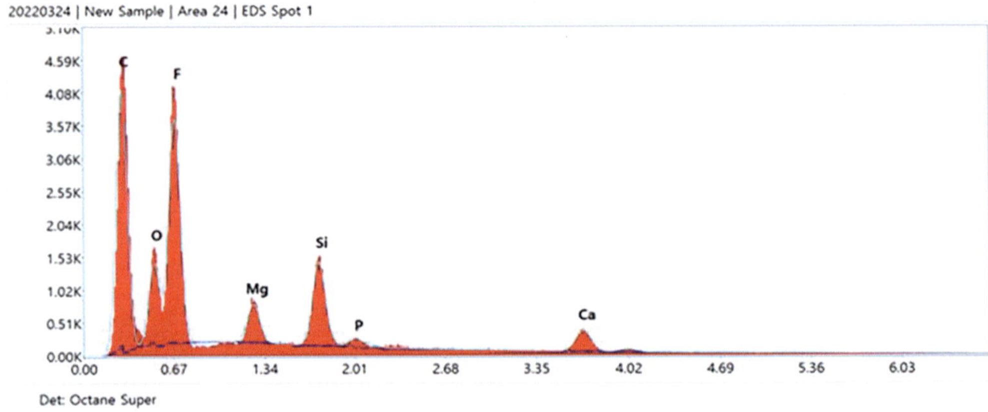

eZAF Quant Result - Analysis Uncertainty: 8.90 %

Element	Weight %	MDL	Atomic %	Net Int.	Error %	R	A	F
C K	58.8	0.77	70.0	2037.9	8.4	0.9343	0.3990	1.0000
O K	12.5	0.55	11.2	660.6	10.2	0.9440	0.3045	1.0000
F K	19.0	0.39	14.3	1876.8	8.4	0.9479	0.4212	1.0000
Mg K	1.5	0.11	0.9	333.4	7.3	0.9583	0.7656	1.0038
Si K	3.9	0.13	2.0	778.5	4.5	0.9643	0.8953	1.0058
P K	0.5	0.13	0.3	86.4	11.0	0.9672	0.9187	1.0083
Ca K	3.7	0.31	1.3	226.6	7.3	0.9799	0.9875	1.0226

Fig. 6.17 EDAX results of product D, where silicone, Ca, Mg, P and other elements were detected

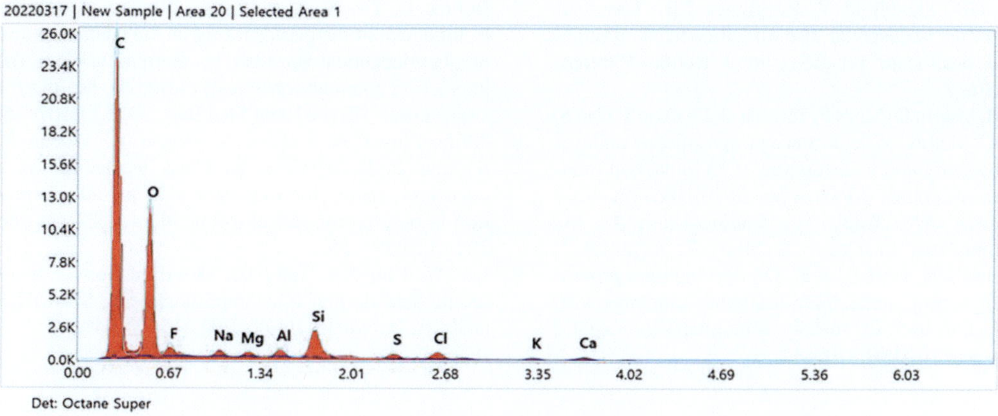

eZAF Quant Result - Analysis Uncertainty: 8.69 %

Element	Weight %	MDL	Atomic %	Net Int.	Error %	R	A	F
C K	67.3	0.11	75.0	5893.4	7.5	0.9401	0.4566	1.0000
O K	26.1	0.09	21.8	2985.8	9.5	0.9491	0.2994	1.0000
F K	1.2	0.07	0.8	219.4	14.4	0.9528	0.3538	1.0000
Na K	0.4	0.04	0.2	148.7	8.7	0.9592	0.6782	1.0021
Mg K	0.3	0.03	0.1	131.6	8.2	0.9623	0.7896	1.0035
Al K	0.4	0.03	0.2	210.5	6.6	0.9652	0.8637	1.0056
Si K	1.8	0.03	0.8	785.6	4.0	0.9679	0.9105	1.0061
S K	0.5	0.04	0.2	172.7	6.1	0.9730	0.9579	1.0129
Cl K	0.8	0.04	0.3	214.5	5.4	0.9753	0.9706	1.0157
K K	0.4	0.06	0.1	65.6	15.1	0.9799	0.9854	1.0282
Ca K	0.8	0.08	0.3	106.9	10.2	0.9821	0.9895	1.0282

Fig. 6.18 EDAX results of product F, where various elements such as Si, Al, Mg, and Ca were detected

is the most commonly detected metal among others [1]. These metals are believed to originate from the grinders or other equipment used during manufacturing.

6.7 Conclusion

HA fillers inevitably contain a certain amount of impurities during the manufacturing process. These impurities vary in size and quantity, depending on the type of HA filler used. The problem lies in the fact that these impurities can clearly trigger immune reactions. Impurities larger than the size at which macrophages phagocytose naturally form giant cells and become factors that can cause foreign body reactions. Therefore, stricter management of impurities is required in the manufacturing process of HA fillers, and the physicians also should have responsibility to choose the safe products [9].

References

1. Langille SE. Particulate matter in injectable drug products. PDA J Pharm Sci Technol. 2013;67:186–200.
2. US Pharmacopeia. U.S. Pharmacopeia and National Formulary. Rockville, MD: The United States Pharmacopeial Convention, Inc.; 2021.
3. Pharmaeuropa. European Pharmacopoeia. Strasbourg: Council of Europe; 2019.

4. Melo GB, Shoenfeld Y, Rodrigues EB. The risks behind the widespread use of siliconized syringes in the healthcare practice. Int J Retina Vitreous. 2021;7:66.
5. Cua M, Martin D, Meza P, Torraca G, Pearson T, Cao S, Yang C. Method to determine syringe silicone oil layer heterogeneity and investigation of its impact on product particle counts. J Pharm Sci. 2020;109:3292–9.
6. Wakankar AA, Wang YJ, Canova-Davis E, Ma S, Schmalzing D, Grieco J, Milby T, Reynolds T, Mazzarella K, Hoff E, et al. On developing a process for conducting extractable-leachable assessment of components used for storage of biopharmaceuticals. J Pharm Sci. 2010;99:2209–18.
7. Bohrer D, Do Nascimento PC, Binotto R, Becker E. Influence of the glass packing on the contamination of pharmaceutical products by aluminium. Part III: interaction container-chemicals during the heating for sterilisation. J Trace Elem Med Biol. 2003;17:107–15.
8. Allmendinger A, Lebouc V, Bonati L, Woehr A, Kishore RSK, Abstiens K. Glass leachables as a nucleation factor for free fatty acid particle formation in biopharmaceutical formulations. J Pharm Sci. 2021;110:785–95.
9. Lee W, Rho NK, Yang EJ. Determination of hyaluronic acid dermal filler impurities using SEM/EDS analysis. Polymers (Basel). 2023;15(7):1649.

Etiology of Delayed Inflammatory Reaction Induced by Hyaluronic Acid Filler

7

Contents

7.1 Introduction

Delayed edema, also known as a delayed inflammatory reaction or delayed-type hypersensitivity reaction, refers to symptoms accompanied by inflammation that occur 2–3 weeks after injection. Interest in this condition has increased worldwide owing to the emergence of the coronavirus disease (COVID-19) pandemic. Systemic changes occur when infected with the COVID-19 virus or when vaccinated, and delayed inflammatory reactions have been reported in individuals who previously received hyaluronic acid fillers. Therefore, it is expected that the patient's condition will have a significant impact; however, the exact cause has not yet been described. This chapter provides a detailed description of possible causes of delayed inflammatory reactions.

7.2 Hyaluronic Acid Filler as a Biomaterial

Hyaluronic acid (HA) fillers are technically foreign substances. Traditionally, tissue expansion procedures involving implant insertion have been frequently performed in the field of plastic surgery. Breast augmentation procedures involve the insertion of breast implants and augmentation rhinoplasty involves the insertion of nasal implants. Furthermore, substances referred to as skin boosters or biostimulators, which are increasingly used recently, also fall into the category of foreign substances. One problem lies in tissue response to these substances. To understand these tissue responses, it is necessary to understand their definitions.

W. Lee, *Advances in Hyaluronic Acid Filler Injections*,
https://doi.org/10.1007/978-981-97-6528-7_7

Definitions:

Inflammatory response: Cellular and tissue reaction to injury.

Immunogenicity: Tendency to induce immune responses.

Biocompatibility: Stable healing process without significant inflammation or irritation.

Generally, the most important factor for an implant to be inserted into the human body is of its biocompatibility, an essential function of the immune system.

When a foreign substance enters the body, it triggers both the innate and the adaptive immunity (Fig. 7.1). Macrophages are one of the most important cells in the process as they phagocytose small foreign substances, but fuse together to form giant macrophages when encountering large foreign substances. And as fibroblasts transform into myofibroblasts, they form fibrous bands. Therefore, a capsule composed of giant cell macrophages and myofibroblasts is formed around the implant.

The wound healing process is divided into several stages. However, these can be broadly categorized into two stages. The first stage is inflammation, and the second stage is healing. During the healing stage, processes such as remodeling, scar formation, and fibrous capsule formation occur. In the inflammatory stage, the cells responsible for foreign body reaction are giant cell macrophages, while myofibroblasts primarily contribute to fibrous capsule formation in the healing stage (Fig. 7.2).

Biomaterials can be categorized into three types. First, living tissues or substances are designed to replace the functions of living tissues or organs that do not show tissue or pharmacological reactions and are inert. Second, there are nonviable materials designed to interact with biological systems and are used as medical devices to replace or supplement damaged organs or tissues. Finally, materials have been developed not only for transplantation but also for diagnosing and treating diseases in the human body. When in contact with biological tissues, blood, or body fluids, these materials do not exhibit biological rejection or toxic reactions, indicating their biocompatibility (Table 7.1).

Biomaterials can be divided into various types depending on the type of polymer material (such as nylon or silicone) and metallic materials (such as titanium). They are classified according to whether the raw materials are natural or synthetic.

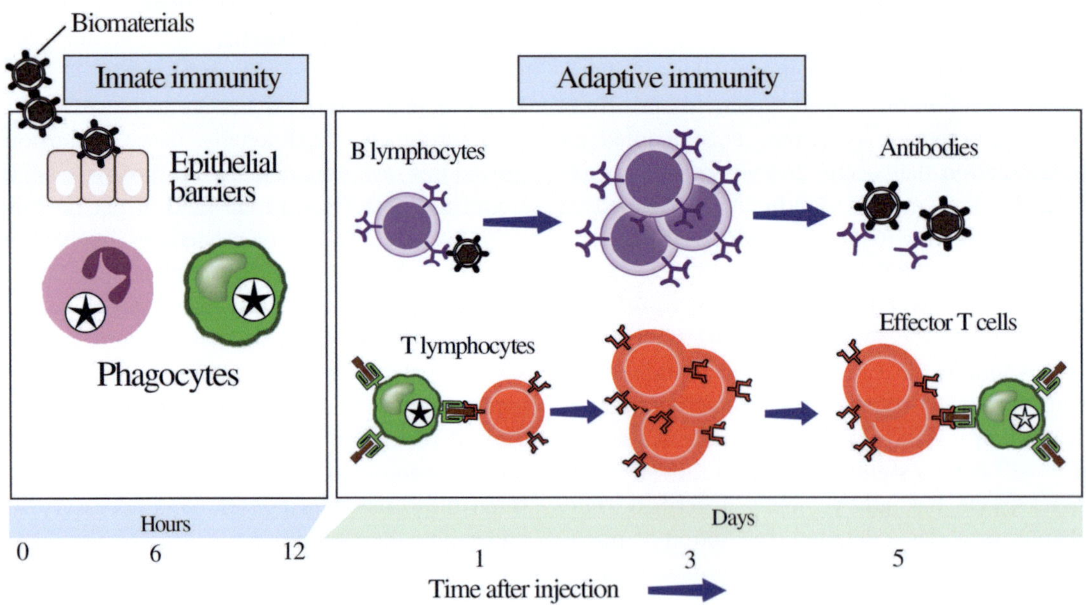

Fig. 7.1 Immune response over time

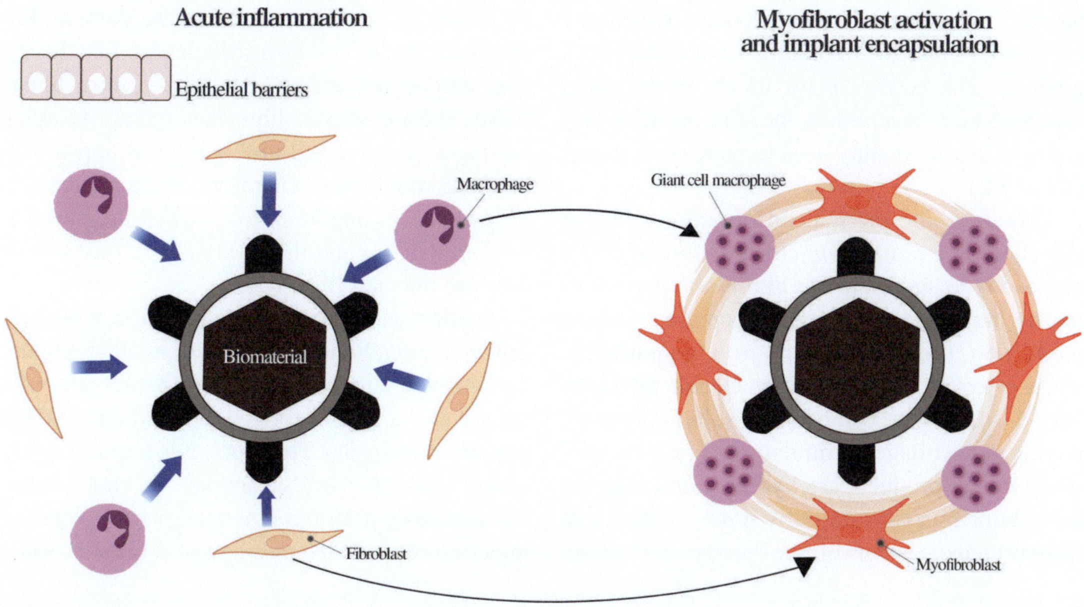

Fig. 7.2 Foreign body reaction by giant cell macrophage and myofibroblast

Table 7.1 Biomaterial classification

Classification		Examples
Material	Polymers	Polyamide (Nylon), acryl polymers, fluorocarbon polymer (Teflon), polyester (Dacron), silicon rubber, polyurethane, hydrogels
	Steel	Stainless steel, cobalt-chrome alloys, titanium alloys
	Ceramic	Alumina, titanium oxides, carbons, hydroxyapatite, calcium phosphate
	Complex material	Carbon-carbon, ceramic-coated metal, carbon-coated material
Raw	Natural	Natural rubber, proteins (collagen, gelatin, fibrinogen), polysaccharides (alginate, chitosan, hyaluronate, cellulose, heparin)
	Synthetic	Polyamide (Nylon), acryl polymers, fluorocarbon polymer (Teflon), polyester (Dacron), silicone rubber, polyurethane
Degradation	Nonabsorbable	Polyamide (Nylon), acryl polymers, fluorocarbon polymer (Teflon), polyester (Dacron), silicone rubber, polyurethane
	Absorbable	Polylactic acid, polyglycolic acid, polycaprolactone, polydioxanone, calcium phosphate

HA is a natural material that normally exists in the human body and belongs to the category of biodegradable materials.

7.3 Skin Boosters (Biostimulators)

To understand the cause of delayed inflammatory reactions of HA fillers, it is helpful to compare the body's reactions to other products. As shown in Table 7.1, there are various types of biomaterials. Various polymeric materials have been used in plastic surgery and dermatology. The most important factor is which layer they target. In other words, HA fillers are mainly used in the subcutaneous fat layers or spaces under the muscles to increase volume. Although various products are also used for injection into subcutaneous fat, HA fillers are most commonly used for volume enhancement because of their ability to dissolve. Skin boosters or biostimulators are products that stimulate fibroblasts in the dermal layer to produce collagen. The term "skin booster" was derived from products developed for injection into the dermal layer of Galderma's products. HA is known for its ability to retain skin moisture. In addition, the skin boosters currently in use are mainly used to increase collagen (Table 7.2).

Therefore, the mechanism of action of these skin boosters remains unclear. Ultimately, the purpose is to stimulate the fibroblasts present in the dermal layer, to thereby increase collagen production. Products used for volume purposes, when injected into the subcutaneous fat layer, have a different mechanism for volume increase that is not collagen-stimulating. For example, when PLLA products are hydrated and injected for volume purposes, initially it may appear that there is an increase in volume, but the mechanism by which PLLA itself increases the volume differs from that of collagen stimulation. The theory that adipocytes themselves, rather than fibroblasts, induce adipose fibrosis and that M2 macrophages are involved in this process appears to be more convincing. Therefore, when using such products, it is important to consider the purpose of the injection and the layers of the face where they are injected (Fig. 7.3).

In addition to the mechanism of action of each product, granuloma formation is another important consideration. As mentioned earlier, HA fillers are also a type of foreign material due to their crosslinking agents. Therefore, it is important that severe foreign body reactions do not occur. Inflammatory reactions that occur when fillers are injected are classified as follows [1] (Table 7.3):

Table 7.2 Biodegradable synthetic polymer products approved for injection applications (South Korea)

Main ingredient	Form	Storage	Reconstitution before use	Products
PLLA	Lyophilized powders	Vial	Yes	SCULPTRA (Galderma, Switzerland)
PDLLA	Lyophilized powders	Vial	Yes	JUVELOOK (VAIM, Korea)
PCL	Gel-form suspension	Pre-filled syringe	No	ELLANSE (AQTIS Medical, The Netherlands) LAFULLEN (Samyang Holdings, Korea)
PDO	Lyophilized powders	Vial	Yes	ULTRACOL (Ultra V, Korea)

PLLA poly L lactic acid, *PDLLA* poly D&L lactic acid, *PCL* polycaprolactone, *PDO* polydioxanone

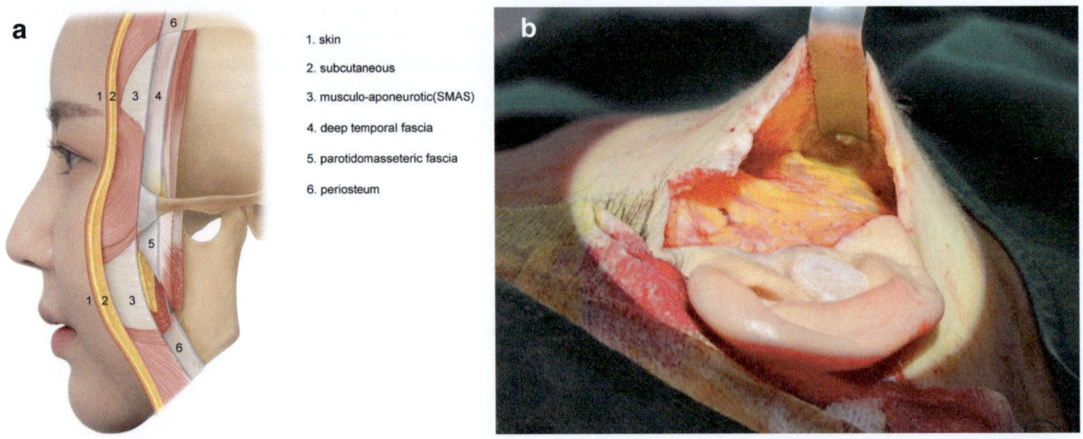

Fig. 7.3 Layers of the skin. (**a**) Schematic diagram. (**b**) Subcutaneous fat layer during conventional face lift operation; when using the product, it is necessary to distinguish whether the injection is intended for the dermal layer or the subcutaneous fat layer and interpret the mechanism of action on the human body

Table 7.3 Foreign body reaction classification (Duranti classification)

Grade I: Slight reaction with a few inflammatory cells
Grade II: Clear inflammatory reaction with one or two giant cells
Grade III: Fibrosis tissue with inflammatory cells, lymphocytes and giant cells
Grade IV: Granuloma with encapsulated implants and clear foreign body reaction

The purpose of a skin booster is believed to be the continuous induction of grade II foreign body reactions. However, depending on the product ingredients, various foreign body reactions may occur in different individuals. It is not an exaggeration to say that the mechanisms of normal and foreign body reactions depend on granulomatous reactions (Fig. 7.4).

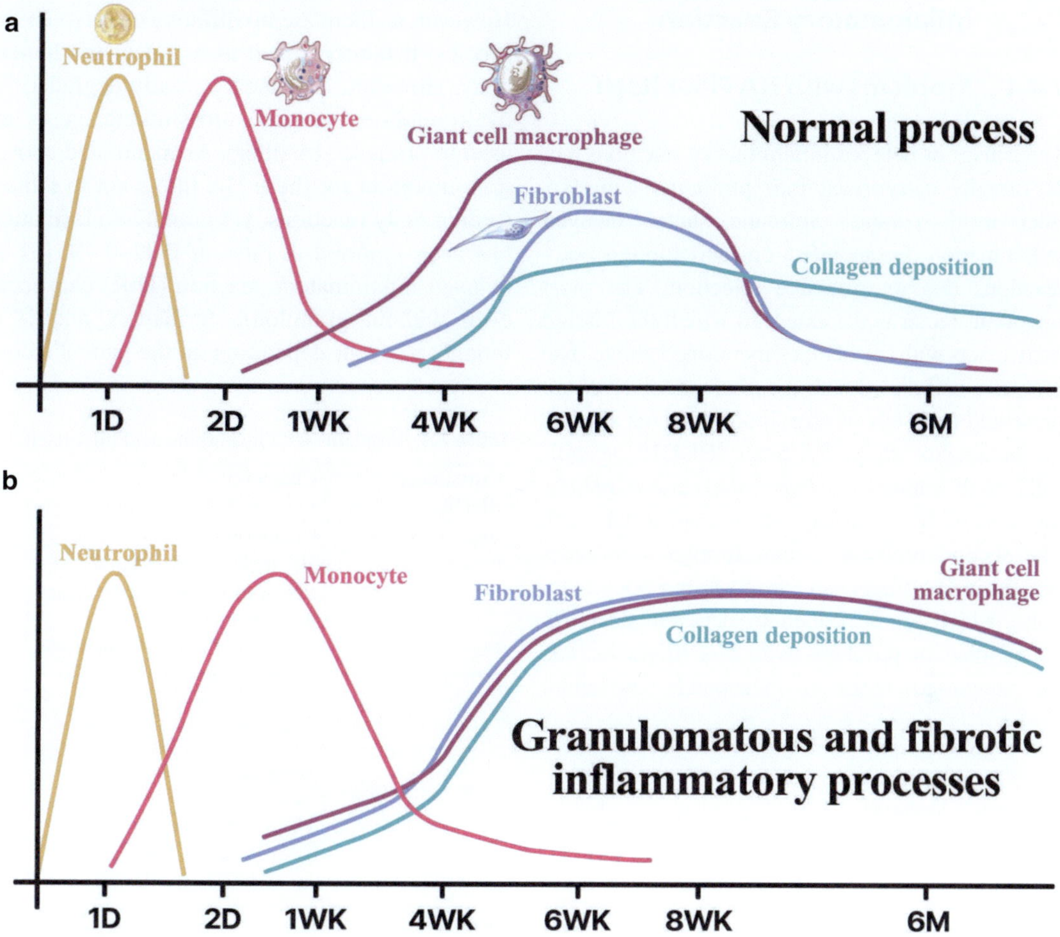

Fig. 7.4 Wound healing process: (**a**) Normal reaction. (**b**) Foreign body reaction

In other words, breast and nasal implants used in plastic surgery correspond to grade IV. However, there have been case reports of HA fillers also inducing granulomas. Several factors have been suggested that are presumed to be directly associated with delayed inflammatory reactions.

7.4 The Etiology of Delayed Inflammatory Reaction

7.4.1 Problems with HA Filler Itself

The causes of delayed inflammatory reactions can be broadly categorized into problems with HA filler itself, patient's immune status, delayed inflammation due to infection, and foreign body reactions due to excessive injection. The most important factor is the extent to which the foreign body reacts with the filler, as mentioned above. The problems associated with the fillers themselves are presented as issues of crosslinking agents such as 1,4 butanediol diglycidyl ether (BDDE), specifically modification of degree (MoD) and crosslinking ratio (CrR), as described in detail in Chap. 5. The second problem is that foreign substances present in HA fillers can cause foreign body reactions, which are described in detail in Chap. 6. Other inherent problems with HA fillers include the suggested range of acceptable molecular weights of the contaminants generated during the manufacturing process (Fig. 7.5). Ultimately, it is important for HA fillers to be clean and not cause foreign body reactions (Table 7.4).

7.4.2 Patient's Immune Status

Hyaluronic acid, which is the raw material for HA fillers, is mostly derived from bacteria. However, as there are no differences between the species, it is recognized as a part of the human body. However, HA itself is easily degraded by hyaluronidase; therefore, crosslinking agents are used to produce HA fillers. As mentioned above, it is important for these HA fillers not to induce foreign body reactions, yet granuloma formation has been reported at rates of 0.02–0.4% [3]. A delayed inflammatory reaction (DIR) can occur even without granuloma formation, and it is thought to occur depending on the patient's con-

Table 7.4 Problems with hyaluronic acid filler itself

Crosslinker BDDE	Chapter 5
Impurities	Chapter 6
Low MW HA	HA induces inflammatory reactions when the molecular weight is low [2]
Manufacturing process	Problem of raw HA, endotoxin, alkaline solution

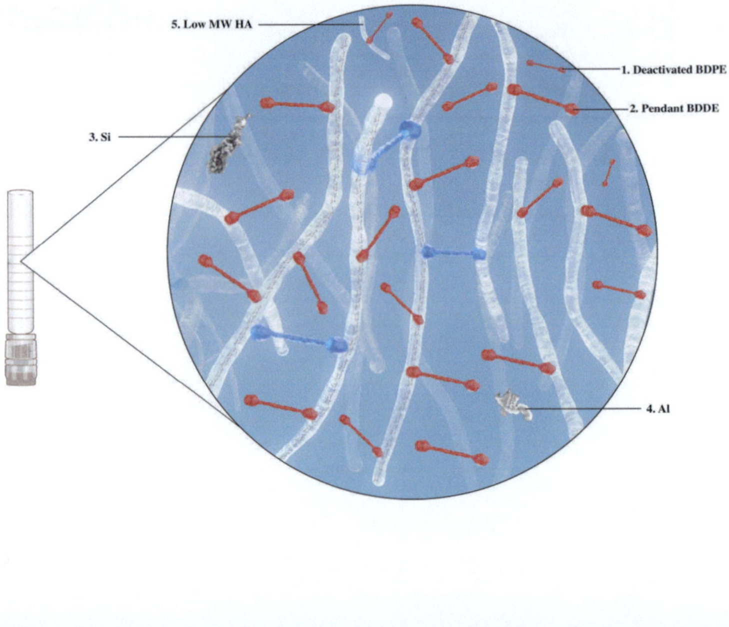

Fig. 7.5 Impurities contained in hyaluronic acid filler

dition. DIR often manifests after symptoms similar to those of the common cold [4]. Therefore, type IV hypersensitivity may occur depending on the patient's condition. Recently, many cases of DIR have been reported during the COVID-19 pandemic, which are believed to be due to increased immune reactions in the presence of viremia or post-vaccination status as well as severe immune reactions caused by virulent bacteria around HA fillers [5]. The spike protein of COVID-19 is thought to act as a trigger, which affects Th1 and CD8+ T cells through the angiotensin-converting enzyme receptor. Therefore, in such cases, treatment with the ACE inhibitor lisinopril is increasing, and DIR is also being treated with steroids and other methods.

7.4.3 Infection

Inflammation is an important factor in all inflammatory processes. Even when injecting HA fillers, aseptic techniques are among the most important factors. However, commensal bacteria can enter the normal skin and coexist with fillers when injected. Therefore, a thorough disinfection is crucial. Although HA filler injection procedures are often perceived as quick, it is essential to remove all makeup and perform thorough disinfection. Apart from disinfection, the patient's previous infection history and filler procedures conducted should be regarded. Chlorhexidine gluconate and isopropanol are the most common recommended disinfectants [6]. Despite the perception that filler procedures are simple, thorough disinfection is necessary and it is crucial to remove the patient's makeup before the procedure.

7.4.4 Bolus Injection

As mentioned previously, HA fillers are created by attaching a crosslinking agent to HA, which naturally exists in the human body. Therefore, it is a substance that can cause foreign body reactions. When foreign substances enter our body, normal macrophages act, and substances that can be phagocytosed are considered to be 5 μm or smaller. If they are larger than 15–20 μm, macrophages cannot engulf them and giant cells are used for phagocytosis [7]. HA fillers, as discussed in Chap. 2, are composed of particles that are mostly of sizes that macrophages cannot engulf. As mentioned earlier, HA fillers cause minimal foreign body reactions according to the Duranti classification. However, the likelihood of foreign body reactions increases when large amounts are injected simultaneously.

7.5 Conclusion

The cause of the delayed inflammatory reaction induced by HA fillers remains unclear. However, DIR is associated with foreign body reactions and causes persistent inflammation around HA fillers. Therefore, the injected HA fillers should be as clean as possible and free of foreign substances. It is also crucial to inject these drugs aseptically and in small amounts to minimize foreign body reactions.

References

1. Lemperle G, Morhenn V, Charrier U. Human histology and persistence of various injectable filler substances for soft tissue augmentation. Aesth Plast Surg. 2003;27(5):354–66; discussion 367. https://doi.org/10.1007/s00266-003-3022-1.
2. Rayahin JE, Buhrman JS, Zhang Y, et al. High and low molecular weight hyaluronic acid differentially influence macrophage activation. ACS Biomater Sci Eng. 2015;1(7):481–93.
3. Lemperle G, Gauthier-Hazan N, Wolters M, et al. Foreign body granulomas after all injectable dermal fillers: part 1. Possible causes. Plast Reconstr Surg. 2009;123(6):1842–63.
4. Turkmani MG, De Boulle K, Philipp-Dormston WG. Delayed hypersensitivity reaction to hyaluronic acid dermal filler following influenza-like illness. Clin Cosmet Investig Dermatol. 2019;12:277–83.
5. Goodman GJ, McDonald CB, Lim A, et al. Making sense of late tissue nodules associated with hyaluronic acid injections. Aesthet Surg J. 2023;43(6):NP438–48.
6. Philipp-Dormston WG, Goodman GJ, De Boulle K, et al. Global approaches to the prevention and management of delayed-onset adverse reactions with hyaluronic acid-based fillers. Plast Reconstr Surg Glob Open. 2020;8(4):e2730.
7. Doshi N, Mitragotri S. Macrophages recognize size and shape of their targets. PLoS One. 2010;5(04):e10051.

8 Vascular Complication: Skin Necrosis Treatment

Contents

8.1 Introduction

Skin necrosis refers to the death of skin tissue that occurs when the arteries supplying the skin are blocked. However, there are also claims that skin necrosis can occur due to compression in addition to embolism. After multiple discussions with various doctors, the general consensus is that skin necrosis is mainly explained by embolism rather than compression, although there is a possibility of skin necrosis due to compression in high-density tissues such as the nose tip. In this chapter, we aim to present the most effective treatment methods available to date.

8.2 Hyaluronidase

One of the reasons why hyaluronic acid (HA) fillers are most commonly used is their ability to be dissolved by hyaluronidase. Hyaluronidase, also known as the hyaluronidase enzyme, is primarily used for hypodermoclysis and to assist the diffusion of other drugs; however, it is currently widely used for dissolving HA fillers. Hyaluronidase has various types, but it is mainly produced in mammalian testes and breaks down the β 1,4 glycosidic bond of HA (Fig. 8.1).

W. Lee, *Advances in Hyaluronic Acid Filler Injections*,
https://doi.org/10.1007/978-981-97-6528-7_8

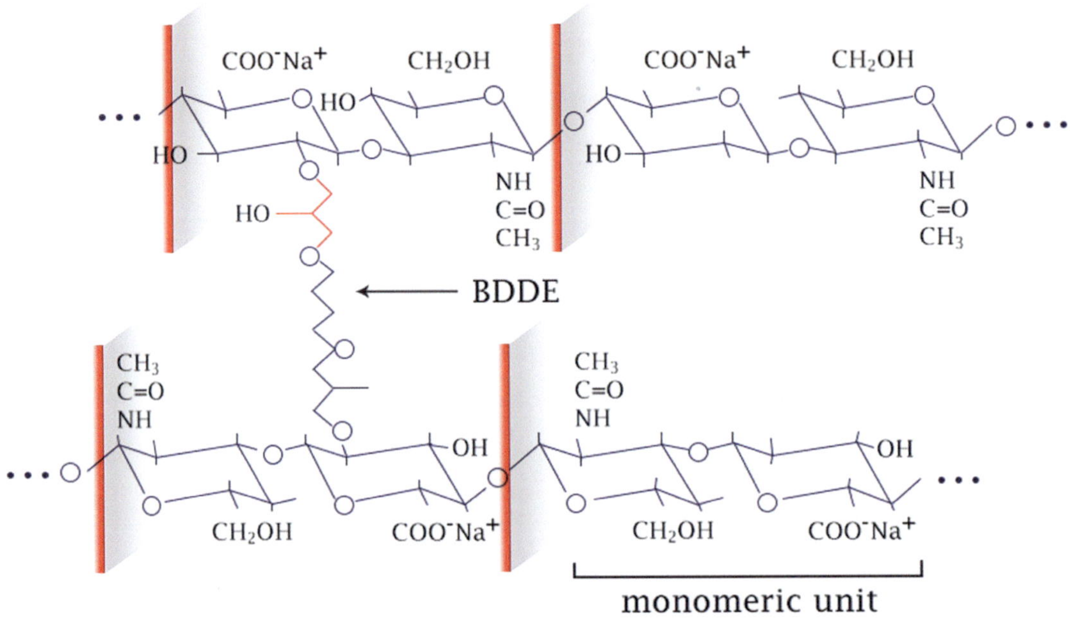

Fig. 8.1 Site where hyaluronidase breaks down hyaluronic acid (red line)

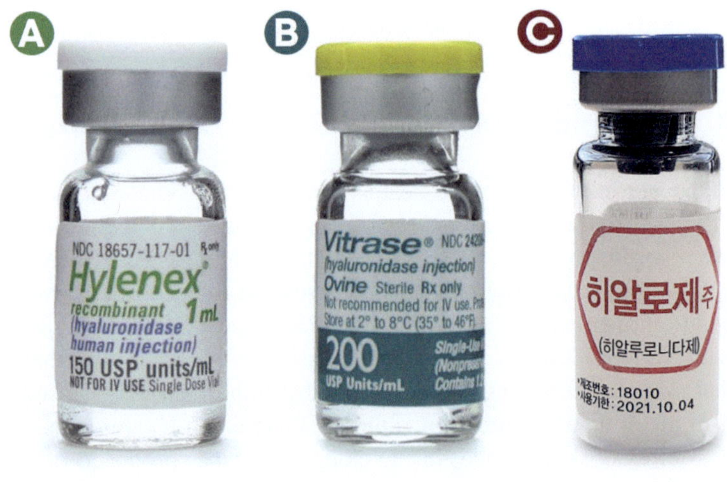

Fig. 8.2 Various types of hyaluronidase (A Hylenex B Vitrase C Hyalorase)

8.3 Types of Hyaluronidase

Hyaluronidase is produced in the animal testes. Vitrase (ISTA Pharmaceuticals) is produced from ovine hyaluronidase and is available at a concentration of 200 USP per vial. Hylenex (Halozyme Therapeutics) is produced from human recombinant hyaluronidase using Chinese hamster ovary cells and is manufactured at a concentration of 150 USP [1]. Hyalorase (Joonghun Pharmaceutical, Seoul, Republic of Korea) consists of 1500 IU and is derived from bovine testes. Additionally, liquid Hirax (BMI, Seoul, Republic of Korea) is also industrially produced from bovine testes (Fig. 8.2). Therefore, the purity of products may vary and allergic reactions may occur as almost all the products are derived from animal testes. The frequency of allergic reactions varies in the literature, with reports ranging from 0.05% to 0.69% [2].

8.4 Five Important Considerations When Using Hyaluronidase Treatment

When skin necrosis occurs due to HA fillers, the first step is to dissolve it with hyaluronidase. However, several factors must be considered before the treatment [3].

The first was the modification of the degree (MoD) of the HA filler used. In other words, HA fillers with a high content of crosslinking agents are more difficult to dissolve. Detailed information on MOD is provided in Chap. 5.

The second consideration is the dosage and efficacy of hyaluronidase. As mentioned above, Hylenex is 150 USP and Hyalorase is 1500 IU. As 1 United States Pharmaceutical (USP) is equivalent to 1 IU, there is a tenfold difference between the two products. However, there may be differences in the purity and other factors during the manufacturing process.

The third consideration is the involvement of the blood vessels. Arteries are interconnected, and when skin necrosis occurs in a certain territory, it should be considered in relation to blood vessels. Skin necrosis caused by injecting HA fillers into the nasolabial folds can extend to the facial, angular, and even the supratrochlear arteries (Fig. 8.3). Hyaluronidase must be injected throughout these territories to achieve the desired effects.

The fourth consideration involves injection of hyaluronidase into the subcutaneous fat layer. The half-life of hyaluronic acid dermal fillers in the bloodstream is approximately 2–3 min, whereas they are known to be within 30 min in the subcutaneous fat layer [4]. Several hypotheses have been proposed to explain this phenomenon. Although the presence of anti-HYAL antibodies in the blood has been hypothesized, they are hardly effective in the bloodstream [5]. Therefore, hyaluronic acid dermal fillers injected into the subcutaneous fat layer can be used for treatment by allowing them to enter the bloodstream. This is the fundamental reason for administering retrobulbar hyaluronidase injections in cases of complications of the eye (Fig. 8.4). The details of the retrobulbar hyaluronidase injection are described in Chap. 9.

The fifth consideration is the need for repeated injections. Considering that the effect lasts for 30 min in the subcutaneous fat layer, it is important to inject into the subcutaneous fat layer multiple times. When blood vessels are blocked by hyaluronic acid fillers, it is difficult for them to dissolve completely at once. Generally, if hyaluronic acid dermal fillers are injected into the subcutaneous layer, and hyaluronidase is injected at the same location, immediate dissolution can be observed. However, in the case of hyaluronic acid fillers that block blood vessels, it is difficult for them to spread from the surrounding blood vessels. However, clinical improvements can be observed when hyaluronic acid dermal fillers are injected in cases of skin necrosis. Therefore, when injecting hyaluronic acid dermal fillers are injected into the subcutaneous fat layer to allow them to spread into the bloodstream, repetitive injections seem to have convincing mechanisms and are important considering that they do not dissolve all at once (Fig. 8.5).

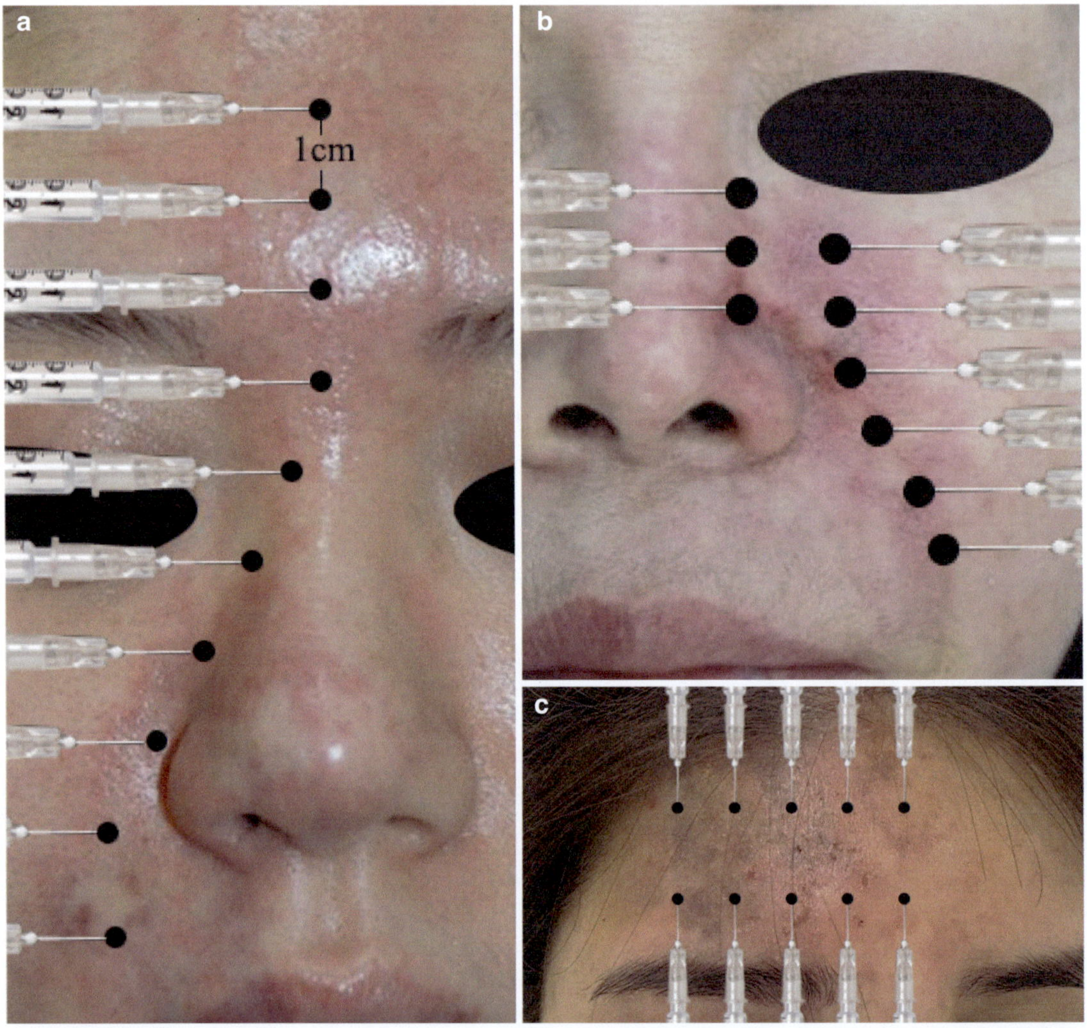

Fig. 8.3 Injection method of hyaluronidase in cases of skin necrosis. (**a**) Hyaluronic acid filler injected for nasolabial fold correction, but skin necrosis occurred in the nasolabial fold area, nose area, and glabella. This indicates the invasion of the facial artery, angular artery, and supratrochlear artery. In this case, injecting hyaluronidase at intervals of 1 cm is recommended, at dosages of at least 100 IU. (**b**) Filler was injected for nasolabial fold correction, and it extended to the nose area. Again, it is recommended to repeat injections at intervals of 1 cm with a minimum dosage of 100 IU each time. (**c**) Forehead augmentation was performed, and the territory of the supratrochlear artery and supraorbital artery were invaded. Each area should ideally be treated with repeated injections of at least 100 IU

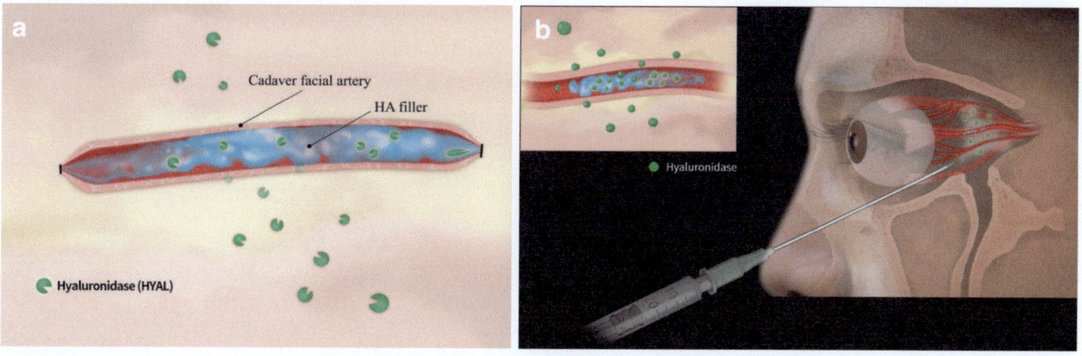

Fig. 8.4 Hyaluronic acid dermal filler subcutaneous injection. Injection into the subcutaneous fat layer for absorption into the bloodstream becomes the basic theory. (**a**) Schematic diagram. (**b**) Retrobulbar hyaluronidase injection

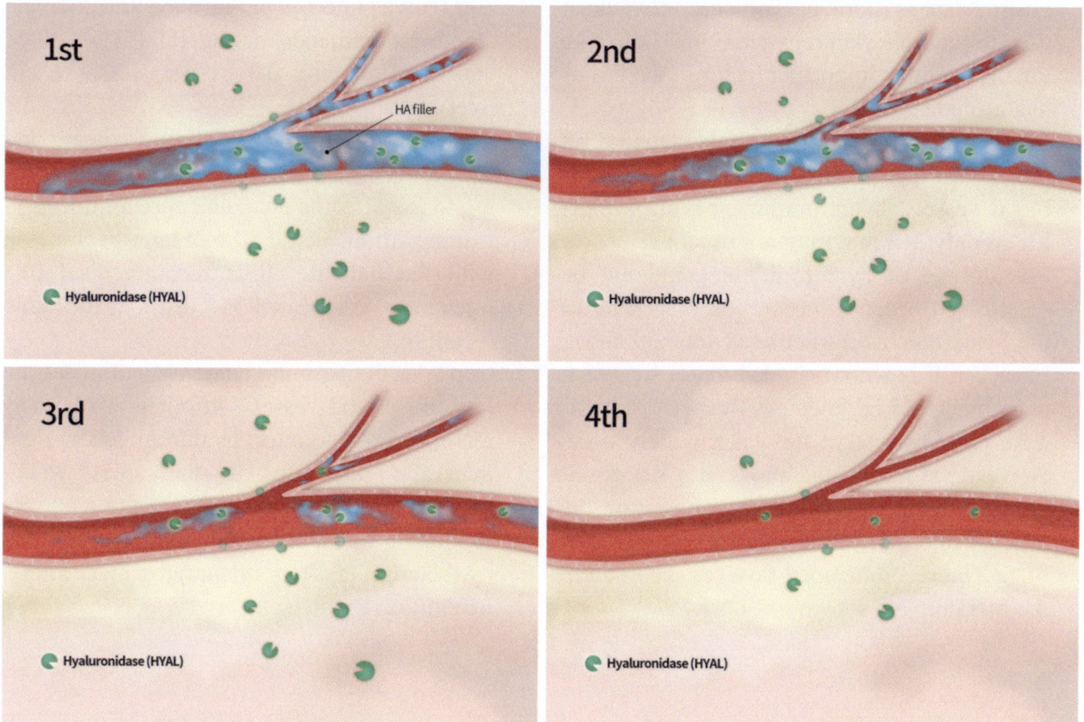

Fig. 8.5 Schematic diagram of repeated injections. The HA fillers in the bloodstream gradually dissolve due to hyaluronidase in the subcutaneous tissue

8.5 Principles of Treatment for Skin Necrosis

1. Prompt treatment. After 48–72 h, hyaluronidase administration might be meaningless. After 72 h, the treatment should be focused on salvaging by high-pressure oxygen (Fig. 8.6), vasodilation, and skin regeneration for the purpose of skin salvage rather than hyaluronidase action. Antibiotics should be administered to prevent secondary infection, and vasodilators should be considered to enhance

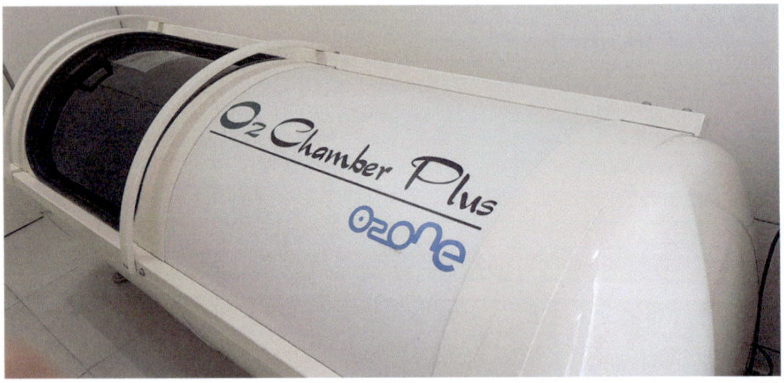

Fig. 8.6 Hyperbaric oxygen therapy machine

the blood supply to the skin. In addition, various substances (pdrn, egf, prp, etc.) have been used to promote skin regeneration. Therefore, time is the most important factor in the use of hyaluronidases.

2. Inject hyaluronidase into the subcutaneous fat rather than the blood vessels. If injected into blood vessels, hyaluronidase, having a half-life of only 2–3 min may not function.
3. The dosage of hyaluronidase could not be determined because the crosslinking state of the hyaluronic acid filler used was unknown. However, it is recommended that a sufficient amount should be injected. Recently, a high-dose pulsed protocol has been widely used. However, as mentioned above, it is not possible to provide an exact dosage based on the efficacy of each hyaluronidase and the type of filler. The recommended dosages recorded in the literature are shown in Fig. 8.7.

   In experimental studies, a minimum of 100 IU was injected per invaded area [6]. The author recommends mixing 1500 IU in a 3 cc vial and injecting 0.3 cc per site at 1 cm intervals.
4. Repeat injections are essential. As mentioned above, inject 750–1500 IU per session according to the affected area, and another injection is to be administered 30 min later to coincide with the half-life. It is recommended that injections be repeated 3–4 times at the same location.
5. Consider the vascular anatomy and inject the invading blood vessels. In other words, it is recommended to inject hyaluronidase at 1 cm intervals, not only in the areas where hyaluronic acid filler is injected to correct nasolabial folds, but also in the areas affected by the angular artery or supratrochlear artery, in addition to the facial artery.

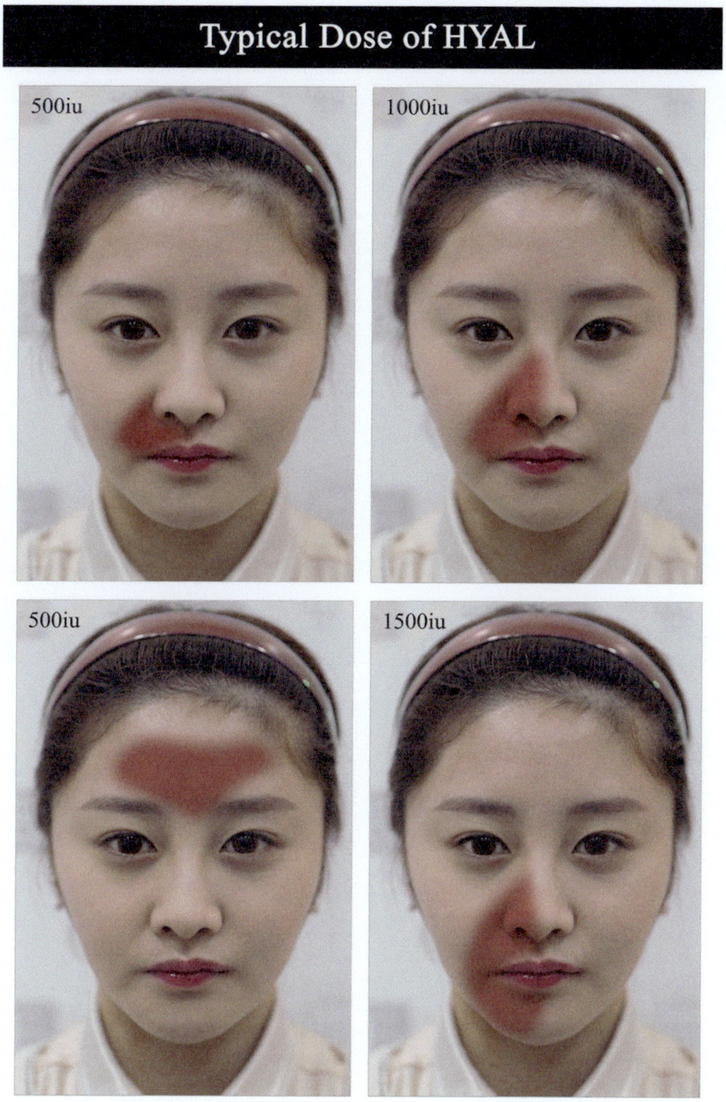

Fig. 8.7 General recommended dosage. The dosage should be considered based on the HA filler MOD and the type of hyaluronidase

References

1. Lee W. Comments on "Hyaluronidase: an overview of its properties, applications, and side effects". Arch Plast Surg. 2020;47(6):626–7. https://doi.org/10.5999/aps.2020.01571.
2. Cavallini M, Gazzola R, Metalla M, Vaienti L. The role of hyaluronidase in the treatment of complications from hyaluronic acid dermal fillers. Aesthet Surg J. 2013;33(8):1167–74. https://doi.org/10.1177/1090820X13511970.
3. Lee W. Five factors to consider before treatment of a hyaluronic acid filler-induced vascular complications. Arch Plast Surg. 2022;49(4):479–81. https://doi.org/10.1055/s-0042-1751102.
4. Zhu GZ, Sun ZS, Liao WX, Cai B, Chen CL, Zheng HH, Zeng L, Luo SK. Efficacy of retrobulbar hyaluronidase injection for vision loss resulting from hyaluronic acid filler embolization. Aesthet Surg J. 2017;38(1):12–22. https://doi.org/10.1093/asj/sjw216.
5. DeLorenzi C. New high dose pulsed hyaluronidase protocol for hyaluronic acid filler vascular adverse events. Aesthet Surg J. 2017;37(7):814–25. https://doi.org/10.1093/asj/sjw251.
6. Lee W, Oh W, Oh SM, Yang EJ. Comparative effectiveness of different interventions of perivascular hyaluronidase. Plast Reconstr Surg. 2020;145(4):957–64. https://doi.org/10.1097/PRS.0000000000006639.

9 Vascular Complication II: Recent Perspectives on Ocular Complications and Treatment Methods

Contents

9.1 Introduction

One of the major adverse effects of fillers is the occurrence of ocular complications. Although ocular complications occur rarely, they can be fatal; therefore prevention becomes crucial. However, there are varying opinions among doctors regarding preventive methods, and treatment methods remain uncertain. In this chapter, I will describe the incidence and pathophysiology of ocular complications induced by hyaluronic acid (HA) fillers, as well as the prevention and treatment methods that I propose.

9.2 Incidence

As of 2024, approximately 60 cases of ocular complications caused by HA fillers have been reported (Table 9.1, Fig. 9.1) [1]. If we included previous cases involving other fillers and fat grafting, the estimated number would be approximately 150 cases [2]. However, some of the reported cases in Table 9.1 may have overlapped; therefore, the actual number of cases was slightly lower. Moreover, it is believed that there are many more cases that have not been reported. Therefore, it is not easy to determine its incidence accurately. However, based on the reported trends, the incidence of ocular complications continues to increase as the use of HA fillers increases. Therefore, further research is required to prevent and treat ocular complications.

The nasal region is the most commonly affected area. The dorsal nasal artery is located on the nose and is directly connected to the ophthalmic artery, making it the most dangerous area. In addition, the supratrochlear artery is located in the forehead, which is also considered a risky area. The nasolabial fold area is relatively

W. Lee, *Advances in Hyaluronic Acid Filler Injections*,
https://doi.org/10.1007/978-981-97-6528-7_9

Table 9.1 Ocular complications induced by HA filler injections

Year	Author	Country	Case	Age	Gender	Ref
2006	Peter	Germany	1	48	M	[3]
2011	Kim	Korea	1	30	F	[4]
2011	Kashkouli	Iran	1	38	F	[5]
2012	Park	Korea	4	26–32	F	[6]
2012	Kwon	Korea	1	20	F	[7]
2013	He	Taiwan	1	52	F	[8]
2014	Oh	Korea	1	33	F	[9]
2014	Carle	USA	1	Late 30	M	[10]
2014	Kim	Korea	1	NA	F	[11]
2014	Kim	Korea	1	23	M	[12]
2014	Chen	China	5	23–45	F	[13]
2014	Lin	China	1	25	F	[14]
2015	Kim	Korea	1	34	F	[15]
2016	Kim	Korea	4	NA	F	[16]
2016	Chen	China	1	22	F	[17]
2016	Hu	China	1	41	F	[18]
2017	Myung	Korea	9	23–62	F	[19]
2017	Lee	Korea	1	25	F	[20]
2018	Thanasarnaksorn	Thailand	6	23–61	F5 M1	[21]
2018	Chen	China	1	31	F	[22]
2018	Sharudin	Malaysia	1	31	F	[23]
2018	Bae	Korea	1	29	F	[24]
2018	Ansari	USA	1	20	F	[25]
2018	Shi	China	1	Early 20	F	[26]
2018	Ramesh	USA	1	23	M	[27]
2019	Yao	China	1	21	F	[28]
2019	Shoughy	Saudi Arabia	1	36	F	[29]
2020	Cen	China	1	22	F	[30]
2020	Akoglu	Turkey	1	37	F	[31]
2020	Cho	Korea	1	51	F	[32]
2020	Kim	Korea	1	23	F	[33]
2020	Downie	USA	2	37, 54	F	[34]
2021	Eldweik	UAE	1	32	F	[35]
2021	Hung	Taiwan	1	31	F	[36]
2021	Lee	Korea	7	23–62	F6, M1	[37]
2022	Wu	China	1	46	F	[38]
2022	Lucaciu	Germany	2	43, 29	F	[39]
2022	Davidova	Germany	1	43	F	[40]
2022	Danks	Australia	1	38	F	[41]
2023	Si	China	1	40	F	[42]
2023	Chung	USA	1	43	F	[43]
2023	Asensio	Spain	1	57	F	[44]

safe as it is supplied by the facial artery, which is a branch of the external carotid artery. Although it is not as directly connected to the internal carotid artery as the dorsal nasal, supratrochlear, and supraorbital arteries, it remains one of the most commonly treated areas and carries a risk of blindness when injected in large amounts.

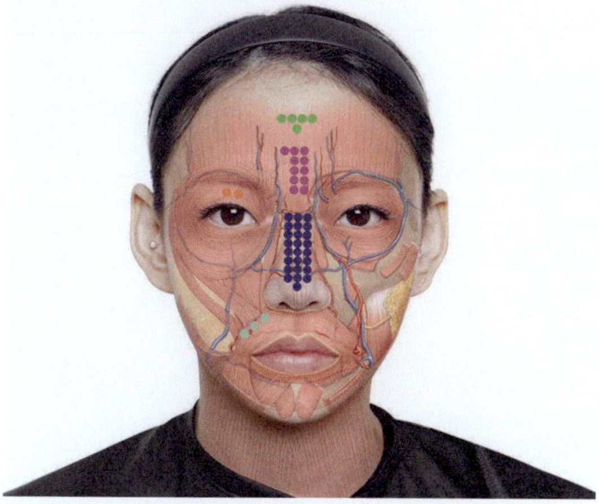

Fig. 9.1 Incidence of ocular complication induced by hyaluronic acid filler

9.3 Pathophysiology

The mechanisms underlying ophthalmic complications caused by HA fillers are well understood [45]. The filler is injected in a retrograde manner through the supratrochlear, supraorbital, and dorsal nasal arteries, which are branches of the internal carotid artery connected to the ophthalmic artery (Fig. 9.2).

Therefore, as mentioned above, when injecting fillers into the nose, the fillers enter through the dorsal nasal artery, and when injecting into the forehead area, they travel through the supratrochlear artery and then follow the ophthalmic artery, leading to an embolism through the central retinal artery (Fig. 9.3).

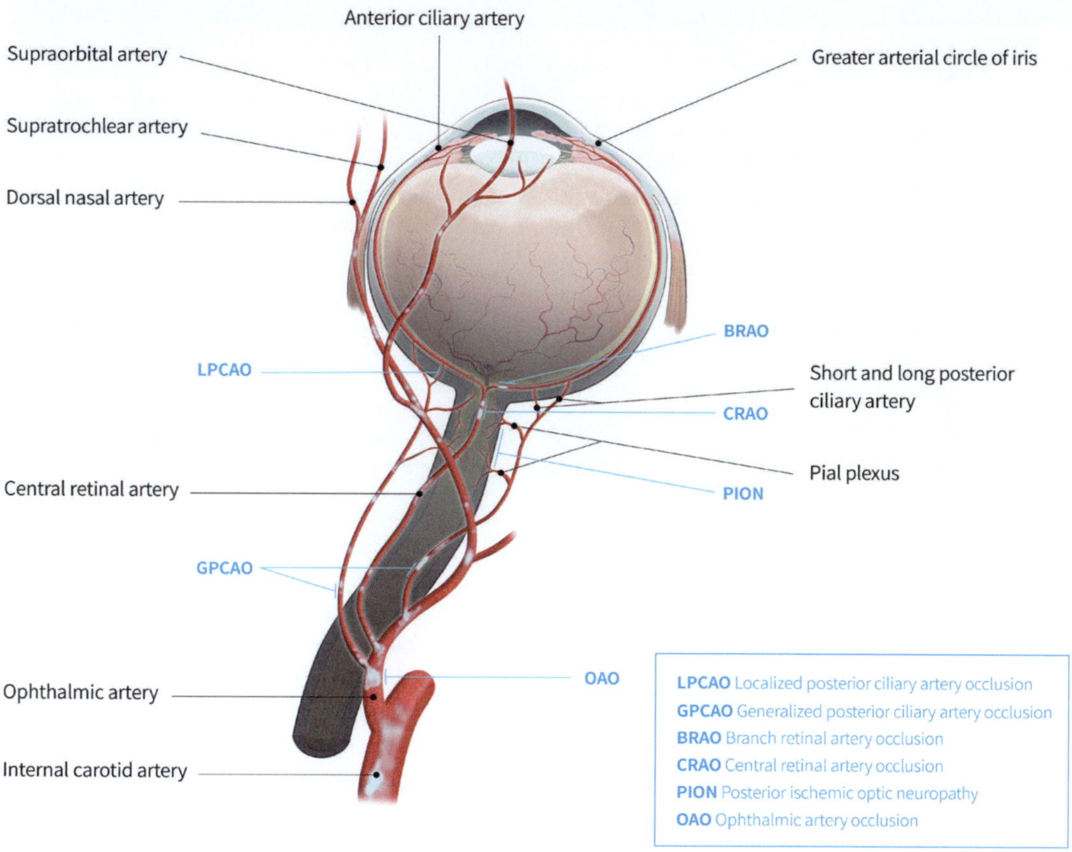

Fig. 9.2 Mechanism of ophthalmic complications caused by hyaluronic acid fillers

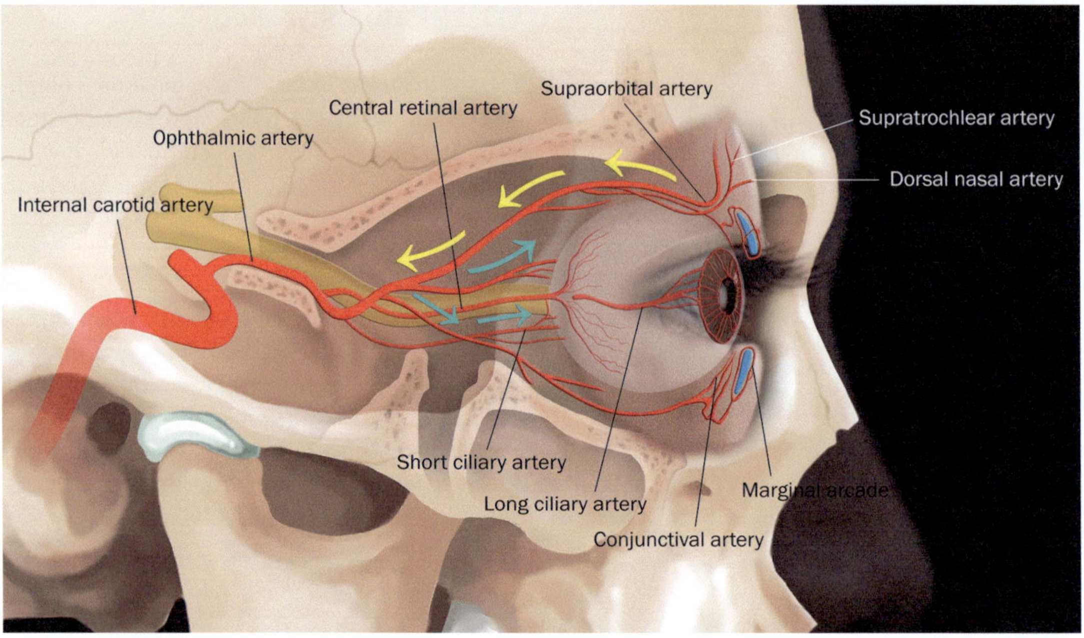

Fig. 9.3 Mechanism of ophthalmic complications caused by hyaluronic acid fillers

This aforementioned mechanism is the most common ophthalmic complication. When injecting fillers into the nasolabial fold area, there is a possibility of the filler entering the eye through the dorsal nasal artery via the facial artery. In addition, when injecting fillers into the temple area, the most convincing mechanism seems to be the entry into the internal carotid artery through the frontal branch of the superficial temporal artery due to anatomical variations. Although anastomosis occurs between the supraorbital artery and the superficial temporal artery (STA), if the filler enters the STA, it is more likely to cause skin necrosis in the hairline area rather than retrograde flow through the supraorbital artery.

9.4 Prevention

Many researchers have proposed methods for preventing ocular complications over the years. However, no study confidently claims that these methods are absolute preventive measures. Although most methods reach a consensus, this chapter describes the ABC technique advocated by the author (Table 9.2) [46].

Table 9.2 ABCs in the prevention of filler-induced ocular complications

(A) Anatomy (Doppler ultrasound)
(A) Aspiration with proper technique
(B) Big cannulas
(C) Compression
(D) Direction of injection
(E) Emergency kit
(F) Filler technique for augmentation or wrinkle correction
(G) Gentle injection of a small amount
(H) History of prior operations or injections

It is universally agreed among all doctors that anatomical knowledge is crucial in prevention. However, there may be variations in the results, and it is important to confirm these findings. To correct glabellar wrinkles, it is essential to confirm the supratrochlear artery before injecting fillers and correct the nasolabial folds, confirming that the facial artery is more important than anything else. The details of ultrasound are described in Chaps. 3 and 4.

The aspiration test is a highly debated preventive method because of its high likelihood of false negatives. The author describes this as an effective method when properly performed in rabbit experiments [47]. First, in vitro experiments were conducted to test cases in which the needle contained air, water, or filler (Fig. 9.4a, b), followed by experiments on the rabbit femoral artery using the same method (Fig. 9.4c). The experimental results suggest that the aspiration test is a useful method unless the needle is filled with a filler. Therefore, the author believes that the first aspiration test is meaningful when fillers are injected using a needle.

Although mentioned several times, the use of a larger-diameter cannula is considered slightly safer. If the tip of the needle enters a blood vessel and the filler is injected, embolism is inevitable. Generally, when considering the average diameter of the supratrochlear artery to be 1 mm, the relative cannula diameter is as shown in Fig. 9.5. Therefore, it is believed that a larger-diameter cannula is slightly safer. The author primarily uses a 21G cannula.

C: The preventive method called "Compression" refers to blocking the artery manually that comes out from the eye and injecting HA filler. In particular, when injecting fillers into the nose or glabella, it is believed that blocking the artery with the hand opposite the injecting hand can prevent ocular complications.

Similarly, the "Direction" is a preventive method that suggests not injecting in the opposite direction of the blood vessels coming out from the eye. The mechanism of ocular complications is that the supratrochlear and dorsal nasal arteries, which branch out from the ophthalmic artery, come out toward the skin, and fillers are injected in the opposite direction; therefore, it is better not to inject in the reverse direction. For example, when injecting fillers into the forehead, injection toward the nose can cause the filler to flow toward the eye if the blood vessels are punctured.

It is essential to have an emergency kit available in clinics. Vascular complications caused by HA fillers have unexpected side effects, and if they occur, they can cause confusion among doctors. Therefore, immediate treatment can be initiated if prepared in advance. Typically, hyaluronidase administration, and, if necessary, timolol, vasodilators, and other available medications is another approach.

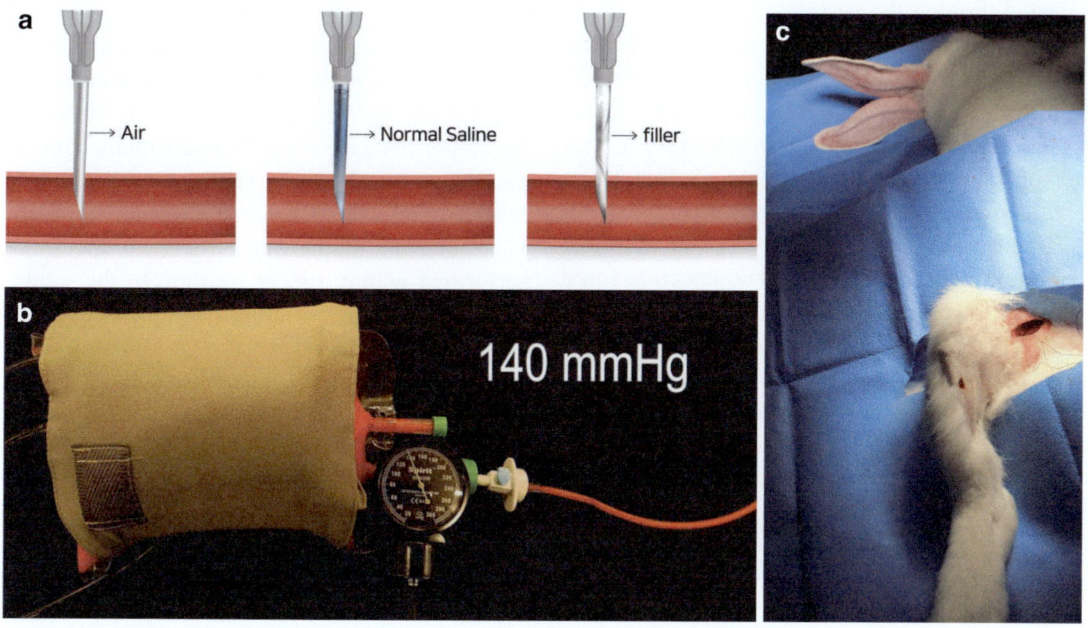

Fig. 9.4 Aspiration test. (**a**) Results are different by needle contained air, water, or filler. (**b**) In vitro. (**c**) In vivo rabbit femoral artery

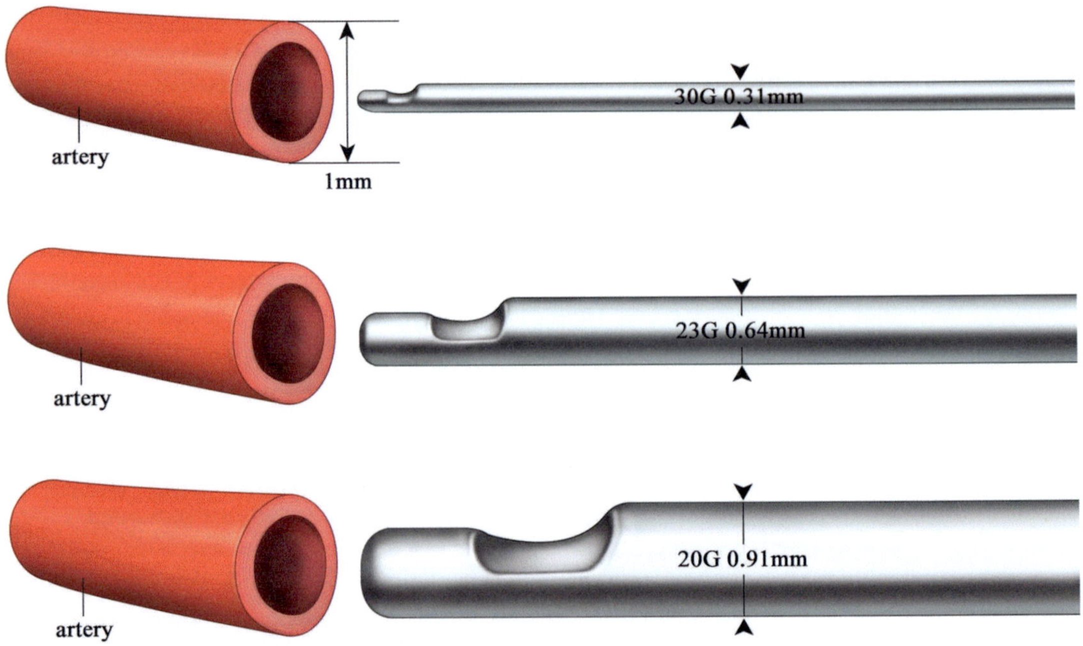

Fig. 9.5 Figure compares the diameter of the supratrochlear artery with the diameter of the cannula

Ocular complications can also occur, depending on the filler technique used. Injecting a bolus is a method that requires caution because once it enters the blood vessels; the filler continues to be injected through the vessels. On the other hand, the linear threading technique involves injecting small amounts at a time, so there is a possibility of necrosis; however, it is considered a safer method for ocular complications because it does not inject the entire volume that can block the ophthalmic artery at once.

Gentle injection is arguably one of the most important injecting methods. The injection force and ejection pressure of HA fillers are significant [48]. Therefore, slow injection minimizes pressure and prevents side effects that may lead to ocular complications, even when the needle tip enters the blood vessel.

Finally, it is essential to ask about previous surgeries or filler injection history before performing the procedure. If there have been previous surgeries or procedures, the likelihood of vascular changes increases, increasing the risk of vascular accidents.

9.5 Treatments

However, there remains much controversy regarding this. According to recent studies, doctors who perform HA filler procedures are advised not to treat the complications themselves, but to refer the patients directly to ophthalmologists through the emergency room [49]. However, the author disagrees with this statement. Time is the most crucial factor. The most critical time point for retinal occlusion is within 4 h [50]. Therefore, the fundamental treatment should be performed within 4 h. In addition to the fundamental treatment methods, the following treatment methods can be performed (Table 9.3).

The fundamental treatment method is the most important aspect of this process. These two methods are being presented as the most important approaches.

9.5.1 Retrobulbar Hyaluronidase Injection

This method involves injecting hyaluronidase into the posterior part of the eyeball. Although this has been suggested in several studies, the main problem that remains is the rebuttal that hyaluronidase cannot penetrate the central retinal artery when it enters the optic nerve; therefore, the treatment remains ineffective. However, a successful case was first recorded in literature from 2017 [51]. Subsequently, the author conducted an experiment on rabbits, creating blindness using HA fillers and injecting hyaluronidase into the posterior part of the eyeball (Fig. 9.6) [52]. The method of injecting hyaluronidase into the posterior part of the eyeball is as follows (Fig. 9.7):

Table 9.3 Suggestive additional treatment of ocular complication induced by HA filler

Treatments	Mechanism
Ocular massage	Sudden drop in intraocular pressure (IOP) with release increases the retinal perfusion
Timolol drops	Suppresses aqueous humor formation, reduces intraocular pressure, and increases perfusion
IV Mannitol, acetzolamide	Medication used in glaucoma to reduce intraocular pressure
Aspirin	Prevents platelet aggregation
Hyperbaric oxygen	Increase oxygen tension and oxygen delivery to ischemic retinal tissue
Steroids	Reduction in vascular endothelial edema

Recent studies have reported cases of vision recovery when hyaluronidase is injected around the eye and then injected again from the peribulbar to the retrobulbar region in the emergency room [41]. Further research is required to confirm this hypothesis. However, at the very least, doctors who inject HA fillers should be aware of this method (Fig. 9.7). To achieve this, it is important to perform and verify posterior intraocular injections in cadaver studies (Fig. 9.8).

9.5.2 Intra-arterial Thrombolytic Therapy (IATT)

Recently, several cases have been reported in China. According to one study, 10 of 24 patients recovered their vision [53]. Furthermore, in a recent study, 26 of 72 patients recovered their

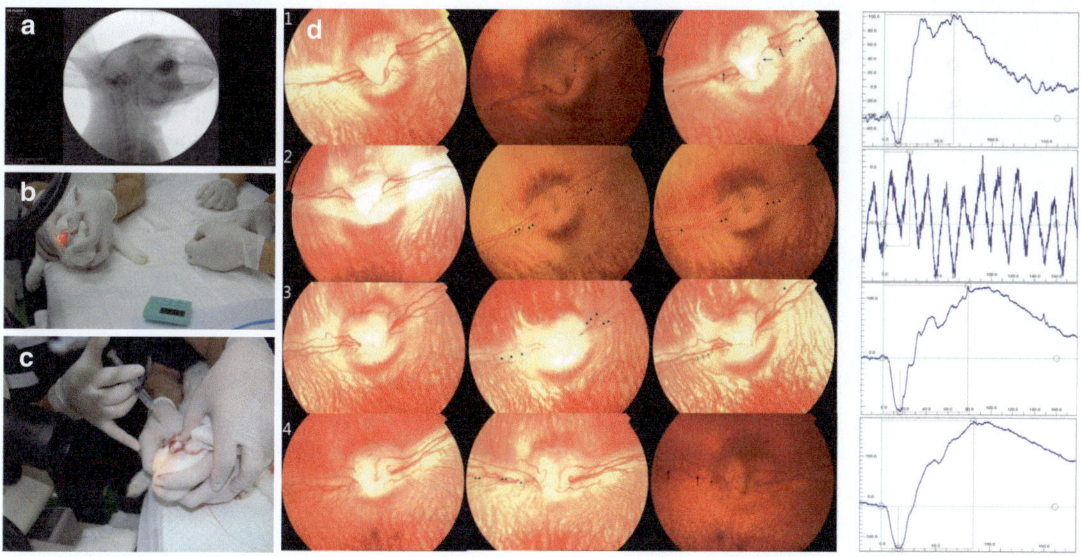

Fig. 9.6 Retrobulbar injection rabbit experiment. (**a**) Angiogram. (**b**) Iatrogenic HA filler injection to ophthalmic artery. (**c**) Retrobulbar hyaluronidase injection. (**d**) Before HA injection (left), after HA filler injection (middle), after hyaluronidase injection and recanalized (right) and electroretinogram (ERG)

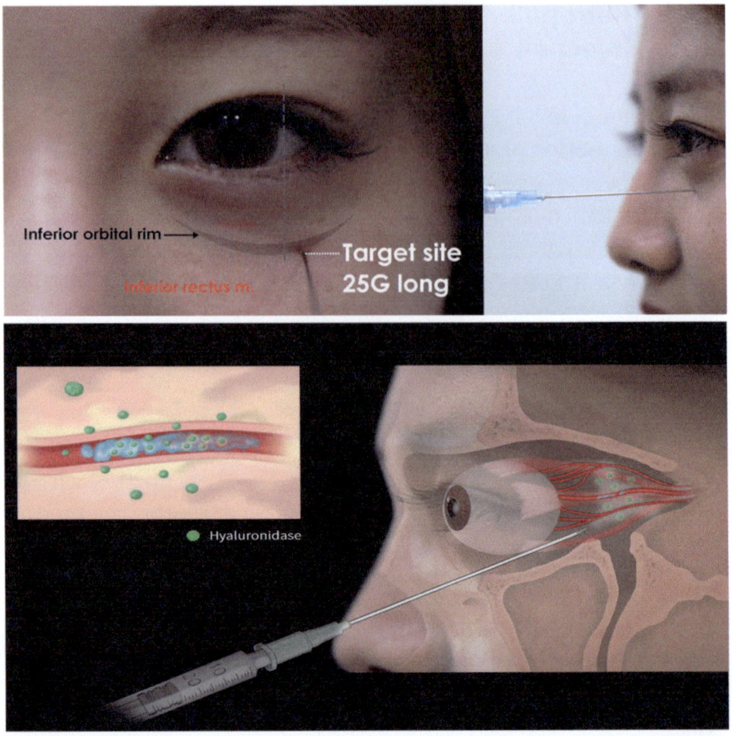

Fig. 9.7 Retrobulbar hyaluronidase injection technique

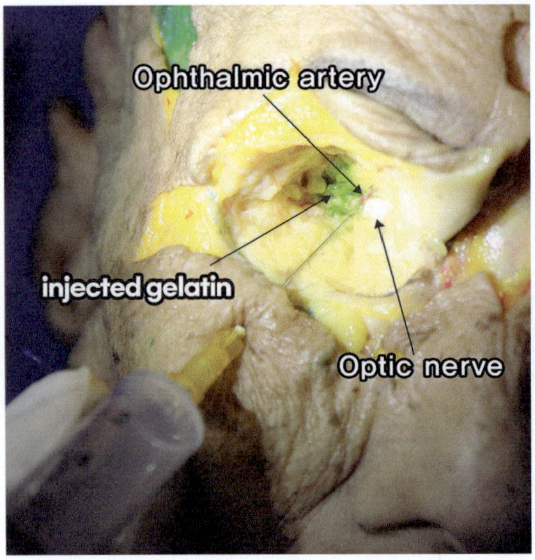

Fig. 9.8 Posterior intraocular injection (cadaver study)

vision [54]. Although there are many cases of recovery, even after a long time has passed since the accident caused by HA fillers and before the IATT, recanalization through the IATT is certainly effective. It has also been confirmed through experiments in rabbits that IATT is effective. The following is an example of a rabbit experiment. First, a microcatheter was inserted into the femoral artery of the rabbits (Fig. 9.8). The progress of the microcatheter reaching the ophthalmic artery through the carotid artery was continuously observed using a C-arm (Fig. 9.9). The No. 2 Lorient HA filler was then diluted with normal saline in a 1:1 ratio and used to block the ophthalmic artery (Figs. 9.10 and 9.11).

To check if the rabbit's ocular blood vessels were blocked, angiograms were taken before and after (Fig. 9.12).

If confirmed by angiogram that the ocular blood vessels were blocked, hyaluronidase was injected after approximately 10 min. After confirming with another angiogram, hyaluronidase was injected again after 10 min (Fig. 9.13). After recanalization of the blood vessels was confirmed, and ERG was performed after 30 min (Fig. 9.14).

Another rabbit was imaged using the same method, which resulted in recanalization (Fig. 9.15).

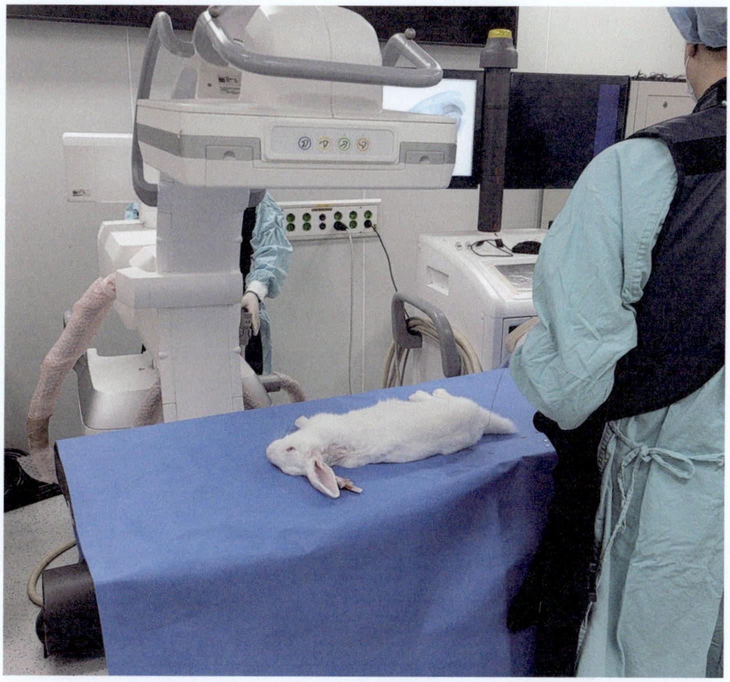

Fig. 9.9 IATT Experiment. A microcatheter inserted into the femoral artery of the rabbit

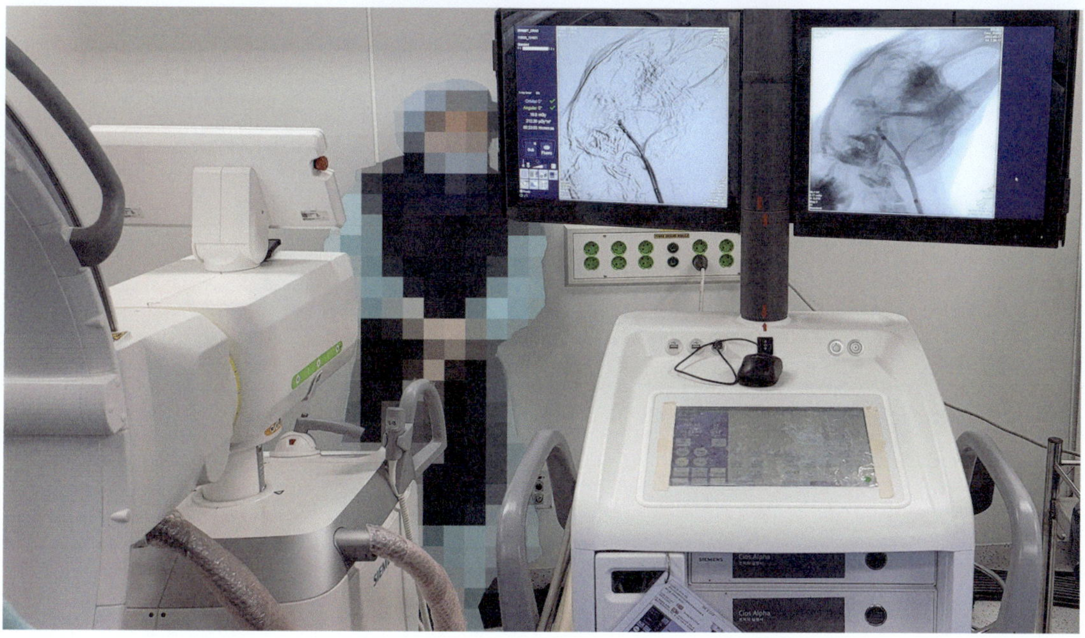

Fig. 9.10 IATT Experiment. C-arm fluoroscopy and angiogram used in the experiment

When complications occur, various considerations should be taken to dissolve the HA fillers. In this rabbit experiment, we chose to block the ocular blood vessels with a filler mixed in a 1:1 ratio of Lorient No. 2. This is because the degradation of HA fillers by hyaluronidase depends on the degree of crosslinking. In other words, fillers with a higher degree of modifica-

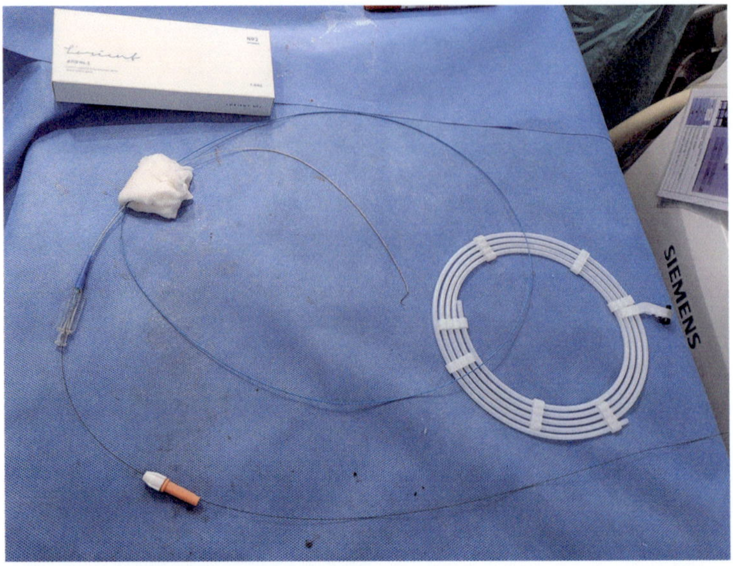

Fig. 9.11 IATT Experiment. Lorient HA filler No. 2 and microcatheter used in the experiment

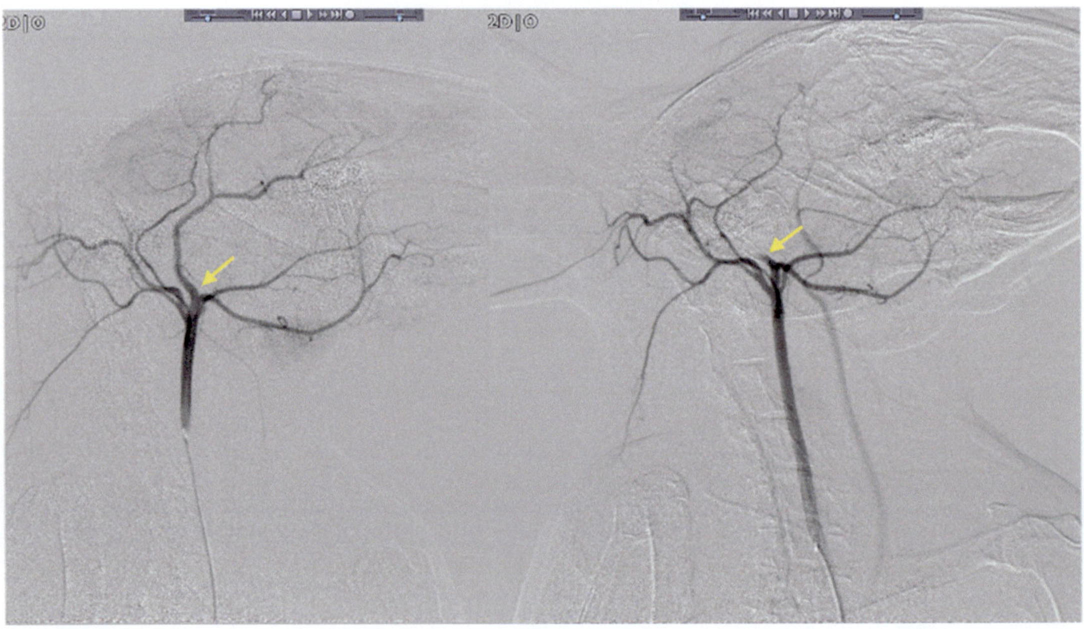

Fig. 9.12 Appearance of the rabbit's ocular blood vessels being blocked (Left: Before filler injection, Right: After filler injection)

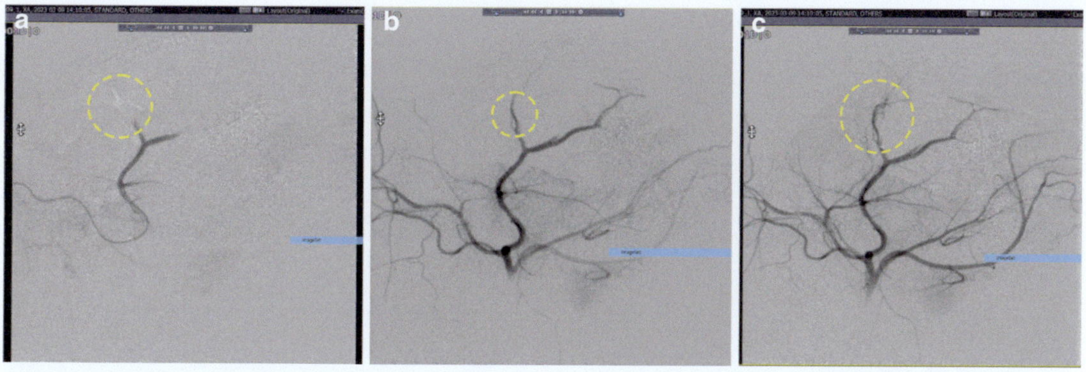

Fig. 9.13 Angiogram taken after injecting hyaluronidase into the ocular artery blocked by HA filler. (**a**) Appearance of blockage by filler. (**b**) After the first injection of hyaluronidase. (**c**) After the second injection of hyaluronidase

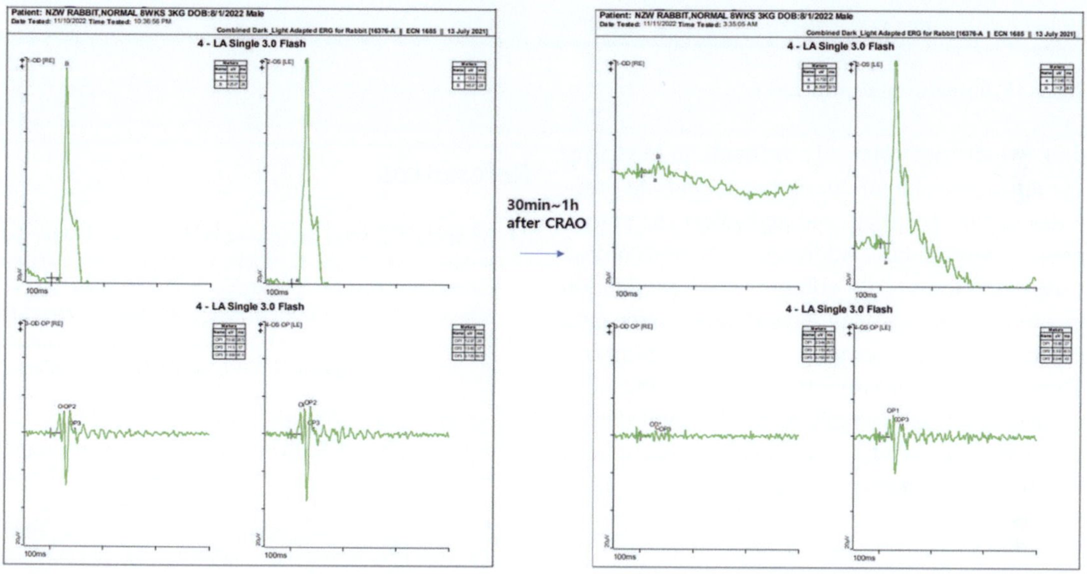

Fig. 9.14 Electroretinogram findings taken after creating central retinal artery occlusion (CRAO) with HA filler

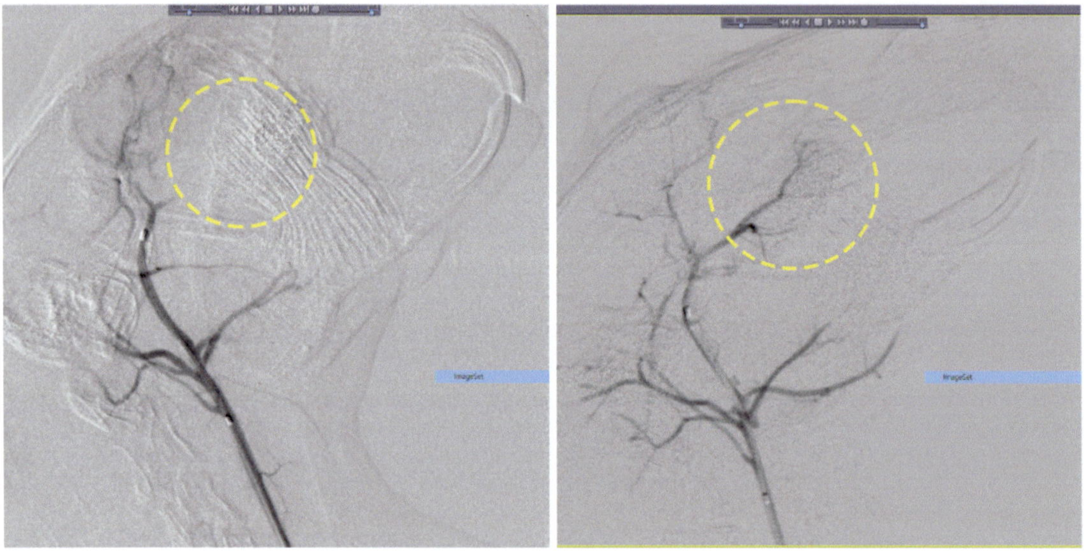

Fig. 9.15 Recanalization with IATT

tion (MoD) are relatively difficult to dissolve. Therefore, it is important to understand the properties of the HA filler used and select the appropriate hyaluronidase. Additionally, hyaluronidase varies in terms of volume and production methods, such as human recombinant, ovine, and bovine origin, varying across countries. Therefore, it is necessary to be aware of the hyaluronidase levels available in the hospital during practice. As of 2024, if complications occur with HA fillers, the author's treatment method is as follows:

1. Contact 911 (emergency medical services)
2. Check pupil reflex and hand movement
3. Prepare 2 cc of 1500 IU of hyaluronidase and perform retrobulbar hyaluronidase injection
4. Perform ocular massage. Administer Timolol to the eye
5. Prepare for transfer and administer hyaluronidase once again if time permits
6. Prepare for transfer. Contact the ophthalmologist at the university hospital and request IATT preparation
7. Continue ocular massage during transfer
8. At the university hospital, perform basic ophthalmic examination and proceed with IATT immediately

References

1. Mortada H, Seraj H, Barasain O, Bamakhrama B, Alhindi NI, Arab K. Ocular complications post-cosmetic periocular hyaluronic acid injections: a systematic review. Aesth Plast Surg. 2022;46(2):760–73.
2. Beleznay K, Carruthers JDA, Humphrey S, Carruthers A, Jones D. Update on avoiding and treating blindness from fillers: a recent review of the world literature. Aesthet Surg J. 2019;39(6):662–74.
3. Peter S, Mennel S. Retinal branch artery occlusion following injection of hyaluronic acid (Restylane). Clin Experiment Ophthalmol. 2006;34(4):363–4.
4. Kim YJ, Kim SS, Song WK, Lee SY, Yoon JS. Ocular ischemia with hypotony after injection of hyaluronic acid gel. Ophthalmic Plast Reconstr Surg. 2011;27(6):e152–5.
5. Kashkouli MB, Heirati A, Pakdel F, Kiavash V. Diplopia after hyaluronic acid gel injection for correction of facial tear trough deformity. Orbit. 2012;31(5):330–1.
6. Park SW, Woo SJ, Park KH, Huh JW, Jung C, Kwon OK. Iatrogenic retinal artery occlusion caused by cosmetic facial filler injections. Am J Ophthalmol. 2012;154(4):653–62.e1.
7. Kwon SG, Hong JW, Roh TS, Kim YS, Rah DK, Kim SS. Ischemic oculomotor nerve palsy and skin necrosis caused by vascular embolization after hyaluronic acid filler injection: a case report. Ann Plast Surg. 2013;71(4):333–4.

8. He MS, Sheu MM, Huang ZL, Tsai CH, Tsai RK. Sudden bilateral vision loss and brain infarction following cosmetic hyaluronic acid injection. JAMA Ophthalmol. 2013;131(9):1234–5.
9. Oh BL, Jung C, Park KH, Hong YJ, Woo SJ. Therapeutic intra-arterial hyaluronidase infusion for ophthalmic artery occlusion following cosmetic facial filler (hyaluronic acid) injection. Neuroophthalmology. 2014;38(1):39–43.
10. Carle MV, Roe R, Novack R, Boyer DS. Cosmetic facial fillers and severe vision loss. JAMA Ophthalmol. 2014;132(5):637–9.
11. Kim SN, Byun DS, Park JH, Han SW, Baik JS, Kim JY, Park JH. Panophthalmoplegia and vision loss after cosmetic nasal dorsum injection. J Clin Neurosci. 2014;21(4):678–80.
12. Kim EG, Eom TK, Kang SJ. Severe visual loss and cerebral infarction after injection of hyaluronic acid gel. J Craniofac Surg. 2014;25(2):684–6.
13. Chen Y, Wang W, Li J, Yu Y, Li L, Lu N. Fundus artery occlusion caused by cosmetic facial injections. Chin Med J. 2014;127(8):1434–7.
14. Lin YC, Chen WC, Liao WC, Hsia TC. Central retinal artery occlusion and brain infarctions after nasal filler injection. QJM. 2015;108(9):731–2.
15. Kim DY, Eom JS, Kim JY. Temporary blindness after an anterior chamber cosmetic filler injection. Aesth Plast Surg. 2015;39(3):428–30.
16. Kim A, Kim SH, Kim HJ, Yang HK, Hwang JM, Kim JS. Ophthalmoplegia as a complication of cosmetic facial filler injection. Acta Ophthalmol. 2016;94(5):e377–9.
17. Chen W, Wu L, Jian XL, Zhang B, Li JY, Qin XL, Yu B. Retinal branch artery embolization following hyaluronic acid injection: a case report. Aesthet Surg J. 2016;36(7):NP219–24.
18. Hu XZ, Hu JY, Wu PS, Yu SB, Kikkawa DO, Lu W. Posterior ciliary artery occlusion caused by hyaluronic acid injections into the forehead: a case report. Medicine (Baltimore). 2016;95(11):e3124.
19. Myung Y, Yim S, Jeong JH, Kim BK, Heo CY, Baek RM, Pak CS. The classification and prognosis of periocular complications related to blindness following cosmetic filler injection. Plast Reconstr Surg. 2017;140(1):61–4.
20. Lee JI, Kang SJ, Sun H. Skin necrosis with oculomotor nerve palsy due to a hyaluronic acid filler injection. Arch Plast Surg. 2017;44(4):340–3.
21. Thanasarnaksorn W, Cotofana S, Rudolph C, Kraisak P, Chanasumon N, Suwanchinda A. Severe vision loss caused by cosmetic filler augmentation: case series with review of cause and therapy. J Cosmet Dermatol. 2018;17(5):712–8.
22. Chen H, Wang H, Yang Z. A case of hyaluronic acid induced blindness with ophthalmoplegia and ptosis. Ophthalmic Plast Reconstr Surg. 2018;34(6):e184–6.
23. Sharudin SN, Ismail MF, Mohamad NF, Vasudevan SK. Complete recovery of filler-induced visual loss following subcutaneous hyaluronidase injection. Neuroophthalmology. 2018;43(2):102–6.
24. Bae IH, Kim MS, Choi H, Na CH, Shin BS. Ischemic oculomotor nerve palsy due to hyaluronic acid filler injection. J Cosmet Dermatol. 2018;17(6):1016–8.
25. Ansari ZA, Choi CJ, Rong AJ, Erickson BP, Tse DT. Ocular and cerebral infarction from periocular filler injection. Orbit. 2019;38(4):322–4.
26. Shi H, Liang LL, Cui ZH. Ophthalmic artery occlusion after cosmetic facial filler injections. JAMA Ophthalmol. 2018;136(6):e180764.
27. Ramesh S, Fiaschetti D, Goldberg RA. Orbital and ocular ischemic syndrome with blindness after facial filler injection. Ophthalmic Plast Reconstr Surg. 2018;34(4):e108–10.
28. Yao B, Shen F, Zhao X, Liu G, Ding Y. Ophthalmic artery occlusion combined with superior sagittal sinus thrombosis caused by hyaluronic acid injection for facial soft tissue augmentation: a case report. Medicine (Baltimore). 2019;98(36):e17048.
29. Shoughy SS. Visual loss following cosmetic facial filler injection. Arq Bras Oftalmol. 2019;82(6):511–3.
30. Cen LP, Wang Y, Li Z. Vision loss after facial injection of hyaluronic acid. Ophthalmology. 2020;127(10):1330.
31. Akoglu G, Ozge G, Eşme P, Erbil H. A case report of episcleral artery embolism caused by hyaluronic acid injection into the malar area. J Cosmet Dermatol. 2020;19(12):3420–2.
32. Cho HH, Ma DJ, Kim MS, Cho IH. Concurrent ophthalmic artery occlusion and optic nerve infarction after cosmetic facial filler. Indian J Ophthalmol. 2020;68(11):2512–4.
33. Kim BJ, You HJ, Jung I, Kim DW. Ophthalmoplegia with skin necrosis after a hyaluronic acid filler injection. J Cosmet Dermatol. 2020;19(6):1307–10.
34. Downie EM, Chen Y, Lucarelli MJ, Burkat CN. Isolated ophthalmoplegia following filler injections to the upper face. Ophthalmic Plast Reconstr Surg. 2020;36(6):e152–4.
35. Eldweik L. Orbital infarction syndrome following hyaluronic acid filler rhinoplasty. Am J Ophthalmol Case Rep. 2021;22:101063.
36. Hung JH, Wang CT, Lee CN, Shieh SJ. Unilateral vision loss after hyaluronic acid injection: a case report. Ann Plast Surg. 2021;86(2S Suppl 1):S127–31.
37. Lee KE, Kim GJ, Sa HS. The clinical spectrum of periorbital vascular complications after facial injection. J Cosmet Dermatol. 2021;20(5):1532–40.
38. Wu Q, Fu Q, Xu X, Zheng C, Zhang J, Chen M. Superselective ophthalmic artery thrombolytic therapy for hyaluronic acid embolization: a case report. Clin Cosmet Investig Dermatol. 2022;15:1459–63.
39. Lucaciu A, Samp PF, Hattingen E, Kestner RI, Davidova P, Kohnen T, Rudolph J, Dietz A, Steinmetz H, Strzelczyk A. Sudden vision loss and neurological deficits after facial hyaluronic acid filler injection. Neurol Res Pract. 2022;4(1):40.
40. Davidova P, Müller M, Wenner Y, König C, Kenikstul N, Kohnen T. Ophthalmic artery occlusion after glabellar hyaluronic acid filler injection. Am J Ophthalmol Case Rep. 2022;26:101407.

41. Danks JJ, Dalgliesh JD, Ayton T. Cosmetic filler blindness: recovery after repeated hyaluronidase injections. Aesthet Surg J. 2022;42(4):411–6.
42. Si M, Wang H. Retinal artery occlusion after facial filler injection in a patient with patent foramen ovale: a case report and literature review. J Int Med Res. 2023;51(9):3000605231194514.
43. Chung CW, Shiuey EJ, Briceño CA, Lee V. Acute diplopia after glabellar hyaluronic acid filler injection. Am J Ophthalmol Case Rep. 2023;31:101860.
44. Asensio-Sánchez VM. Central retinal artery occlusion following facial injection of hyaluronic acid. Arch Soc Esp Oftalmol (Engl Ed). 2023;98(7):410–2.
45. Cho KH, Dalla Pozza E, Toth G, Bassiri Gharb B, Zins JE. Pathophysiology study of filler-induced blindness. Aesthet Surg J. 2019;39(1):96–106.
46. Lee W. Prevention of hyaluronic acid filler-induced blindness. Dermatol Ther. 2020;33(4):e13657.
47. Moon HJ, Lee W, Kim JS, Yang EJ, Sundaram H. Aspiration revisited: prospective evaluation of a physiologically pressurized model with animal correlation and broader applicability to filler complications. Aesthet Surg J. 2021;41(8):NP1073–83.
48. Lee Y, Oh SM, Lee W, Yang EJ. Comparison of hyaluronic acid filler ejection pressure with injection force for safe filler injection. J Cosmet Dermatol. 2021;20(5):1551–6.
49. Walker L, Convery C, Davies E, Murray G, Croasdell B. Consensus opinion for the management of soft tissue filler induced vision loss. J Clin Aesthet Dermatol. 2021;14(12):E84–94.
50. Hayreh SS, Zimmerman MB, Kimura A, Sanon A. Central retinal artery occlusion. Retinal survival time. Exp Eye Res. 2004;78(3):723–36. https://doi.org/10.1016/s0014-4835(03)00214-8.
51. Chesnut C. Restoration of visual loss with retrobulbar hyaluronidase injection after hyaluronic acid filler. Dermatologic Surg. 2018;44(3):435–7.
52. Lee W, Oh W, Ko HS, Lee SY, Kim KW, Yang EJ. Effectiveness of retrobulbar hyaluronidase injection in an iatrogenic blindness rabbit model using hyaluronic acid filler injection. Plast Reconstr Surg. 2019;144(1):137–43.
53. Zhang LX, Lai LY, Zhou GW, Liang LM, Zhou YC, Bai XY, Dai Q, Yu YT, Tang WQ, Chen ML. Evaluation of intraarterial thrombolysis in treatment of cosmetic facial filler-related ophthalmic artery occlusion. Plast Reconstr Surg. 2020;145(1):42e–50.
54. Wang Y, Li Q, Ye Y, Zhang J, Shen H, Zhou Y, Zhou C, Yu Y, Xiong B. Intraarterial thrombolytic treatment for visual deficits caused by hyaluronic acid filler: efficacy, safety, and prognostic factors. Plast Reconstr Surg. 2023;152(6):1226–33.

MIX
Papier aus verantwortungsvollen Quellen
Paper from responsible sources
FSC® C105338

If you have any concerns about our products,
you can contact us on
ProductSafety@springernature.com

In case Publisher is established outside the EU,
the EU authorized representative is:
Springer Nature Customer Service Center GmbH
Europaplatz 3, 69115 Heidelberg, Germany

Printed by Libri Plureos GmbH
in Hamburg, Germany